T0212431

Disruptive Healthcare Provider Behavior

Rade B. Vukmir

Disruptive Healthcare Provider Behavior

An Evidence-Based Guide

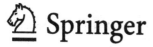 Springer

Rade B. Vukmir, MD, JD
President
Critical Care Medicine Associates
Sewickley, PA, USA

Professor Adjunct
Emergency Medicine
Temple University School of Medicine
Clinical Campus
Pittsburgh, PA, USA

ISBN 978-3-319-27922-0   ISBN 978-3-319-27924-4   (eBook)
DOI 10.1007/978-3-319-27924-4

Library of Congress Control Number: 2016930304

Springer Cham Heidelberg New York Dordrecht London

Springer International Publishing AG Switzerland is part of Springer
Science+Business Media (www.springer.com)

Preface

Disruptive provider behavior is perhaps one of the most complicated areas of medical practice management and hospital administration. The scope of research into this topic has expanded considerably to involve all members of the health-care team, including providers and administrators. The analysis has begun to focus on patient care and quality of life in the health-care workplace, rather than just the effects on an individual or group. As such, approaches toward intervention have shifted from corrective actions targeting the individual to education and proactive intervention that strives to improve the overall system.

This book addresses the theory of disruptive behavior theory, how this behavior is experienced, at-risk groups and situations, regulatory influence, and strategies directed at intervention and improvement. Finally, a set of illustrative case scenarios, including situational analysis and action plans, is presented.

Sewickley, PA, USA   Rade B. Vukmir

Executive Summary

The study of disruptive behavior among health-care providers is based on a multidisciplinary approach emphasizing a comprehensive identification, education, and remediation strategy. The search identified approximately 90 articles published over the past 35 years that reported substantive qualitative and quantitative scientific data and recommendations on this topic.

Here, disruptive provider behavior is defined, its etiology is explored, and it is profiled according to location and specialty correlates. The complex nursing interface and residency training correlates also are analyzed. Most importantly, the effects on patient safety and care quality are reported. In addition, the impact of policies on the economic and legal aspects of the health-care delivery process is evaluated. Lastly, the management interface, interventional strategies, and educational approaches regarding the disruptive behavior dilemma are discussed.

Disruptive provider behavior is a complex, multifaceted problem whose solution requires cooperation among physicians, nurses, and administrators to ensure care quality and patient safety. At the same time, investment of time and effort in a facility's staff has direct benefits in reducing absenteeism and employee turnover, as well as indirect benefits that accrue directly to the patient, as staff performance is improved as well.

Contents

Chapter 1
Introduction

The disruptive health-care provider is not a concept of modern medicine; indeed his or her presence has been documented for well over 100 years [1]. However, although this type of behavior has been noted since ancient times, the term *disruptive* was added only recently as a label. The negative consequences of disruptive conduct by health-care providers are well described by numerous authorities, who posit that this behavior threatens the facility's image, staff morale, finances, and patient quality of care. Therefore, it is essential for hospital leaders to address this issue early on to ensure the pursuit of the hospital's mission and to establish confidence in the facility's operational and business activities and goals.

A disruptive physician may alienate staff, divert patients, and increase the risk of subsequent medical malpractice litigation [2]. The key to managing this type of situation is to develop and execute an effective strategy to confront and address the issue early and definitively and to apply standards universally throughout the institution to all involved parties.

Likewise, disruptive behavior may have a significant adverse impact on the health-care delivery system, potentially affecting patient safety and quality of care [3]. Interestingly, disruptive behavior occurs throughout all the disciplines in the health-care delivery chain: not just among physicians and nurses but also among other staff, including paraprofessional and administrative personnel. This conduct distills down to a level of frustration that may impede communication and collaboration, resulting in avoidable medical errors and adverse events.

© Springer International Publishing Switzerland 2016   1
R.B. Vukmir, *Disruptive Healthcare Provider Behavior*,
DOI 10.1007/978-3-319-27924-4_1

Effective intervention is targeted toward identifying the provocateurs of disruptive behavior to tailor appropriate educational and training programs to improve communication among members of the health-care team. An important caveat is that the term *disruptive health-care provider* should not be applied to a well-intentioned team partner who has valid concerns about the health-care delivery system. It is easy to label a provider as "disruptive" even though his or her concerns are indeed well founded.

One of the earliest descriptions of an organized, systematic approach for addressing disruptive behavior was offered by Linney [4] in 1997. Today's rapidly changing health-care environment makes confronting this problem even more essential. The key is to have in place clearly stated, explicit expectations and guidelines for physician behavior. Policies, procedures, and an operational context should be instituted based on these rules to help steer deviations to conventional standards and finally toward the direction of constructive solutions.

Although the concept of disruptive behavior historically focused on personnel with direct patient contact, typically physicians and nurses, a preeminent research group reported a broader problem [5], describing a more pervasive pattern of behavior involving the entire care spectrum, from ancillary support staff to upper-level administrators. This conduct is poorly quantifiable and apparently unnoticed by patients, yet it still has an adverse impact on the flow of patient care. Therefore, the desired culture of safety and comfort can be achieved by involving all health-care staff in educational programs, individualized coaching, and efforts to confront systemic frustrations that may invite and, in some cases, perpetuate the undesirable behavior.

The actual incidence of these disruptive behaviors is relatively small; however, they may have a significant impact on the health-care system. Conduct such as this may increase workplace stress, create a poor work environment, and contribute to dysfunctional teams. Moreover, Swiggart et al. [6] suggested that disruptive physician behavior may worsen the quality of patient care and result in increased medical malpractice litigation. They cited both internal and external factors that affect the physician's ability to cope with workplace stressors, which may in turn perpetuate this behavior.

References

1. Piper LE. Addressing the phenomenon of disruptive physician behavior. Health Care Manag. 2003;22(4):335–9.
2. Kissoon N, Lapenta S, Armstrong G. Diagnosis and therapy for the disruptive physician. Physician Exec. 2002;28(1):54–8.
3. Rosenstein AH, O'Daniel M. Managing disruptive physician behavior: impact on staff relationships and patient care. Neurology. 2008;70(17):1564–70.
4. Linney BJ. Confronting the disruptive physician. Physician Exec. 1997;23(7):55–8.
5. Zimmerman T, Amori G. The silent organizational pathology of insidious intimidation. J Healthcare Risk Manag. 2011; 30(3):5–6, 8–15.
6. Swiggart WH, Dewey CM, Hickson GB, Finlayson AJ, Spickard WA. A plan for identification, treatment and remediation of disruptive behaviors in physicians. Front Health Serv Manage. 2009;25(4):3–11.

Chapter 2
Scope of the Problem

It has been suggested that the medical community has made significant strides with regard to high-profile areas of provider impairment with obvious external manifestations, such as substance abuse, mental illness, and drug and/or alcohol dependence. However, dealing with disruptive behavior in the health-care arena, which is more nuanced, has posed a significant challenge beyond just discovery. In a broad-brush description, Veltman [1] called disruptive practitioner behavior "contentious, threatening, unreachable, insulting and frequently litigious" and stated that these providers "will not play by the rules" and do not "have the ability to relate or work well with others" [1]. However, this analysis may be too simplistic, as coworker interaction and certainly other providers often are major drivers as well. Thus, it has matured far past the physician-centered, single-focus template.

The most significant behavioral problems tend to surface during routine, periodic evaluation times and typically are associated with the medical staff reappointment time frame [2]. The practitioners being evaluated and/or reappointed often have different strengths and weaknesses of which the evaluators may not be aware, resulting in an unfavorable mix of staff opinion. Therefore, it is critical to provide adequate training, orientation, and senior-level expertise to manage this difficult task.

The key then is to use an evidence-based framework to develop an organizational approach that promotes a healthy, positive work environment that is safe for patients and

© Springer International Publishing Switzerland 2016   5
R.B. Vukmir, *Disruptive Healthcare Provider Behavior*,
DOI 10.1007/978-3-319-27924-4_2

providers alike [3]. This atmosphere will enable the staff to focus on delivering high-quality, cost-effective, and personally satisfying care rather than wasting additional time and emotional energy on reacting to conflict.

A crucial task is to delineate, in a goal-oriented fashion, the various types of dysfunction that may occur among health-care professionals in the workplace, which will provide a framework for analysis. Once the behaviors are defined, they can be monitored, tracked, and analyzed for trends. The following definitions for disruptive physicians are offered based on conduct: The *incompetent* physician lacks the skill, training, experience, or expertise to capably and consistently care for patients. The *impaired* physician normally is competent but is transiently or persistently limited in his or her ability to deliver care by a medical or psychological condition, the use of, abuse of, or dependence on a substance or other intoxicant. Lastly, the *disruptive* physician is competent and is not impaired yet has an interactive style that substantially limits the effectiveness of his or her care (Table 2.1).

The term *disruptive physician* is now in vogue, appearing in written hospital bylaws and described by numerous organized medical bodies, societies, and external regulatory agencies [4]. However, a clear potential exists for its misuse, emphasizing the negative aspect of this pejorative term. Some physicians who have potentially crossed boundaries early in the process may express concern for quality only after their behavior has come under scrutiny and has been labeled as disruptive.

On the other hand, physicians who raise quality concerns with good intentions may inappropriately be targeted as "disruptive" by hospital administration. Whereas the legal system

TABLE 2.1. Description of physician dysfunction.

Term	Definition
Incompetent	Lacks skill in providing consistent care
Impaired	Transiently limited based on medical, psychiatric condition, or substance use
Disruptive	Competent but with limited operational style

discourages the behavior of the former group, it does offer some protected class status in limited circumstances for the latter. Hospitals and medical facilities are given a very wide berth in presiding over their staff's regulatory issues.

Historically, the legal system has had little interest in addressing quality issues in this arena at the hospital level. Its focus, rather, is to question on a procedural level whether the medical staff bylaws were followed uniformly in physician disciplinary proceedings, not necessarily whether they were fair or unfair in substance. The judicial predisposition inferred from case law precedent is to leave this type of decision-making to the individual hospital or facility.

Zbar et al. [4] described several steps in a comprehensive approach to addressing the disruptive behavior phenomenon. First, the physician should be intimately familiar with the medical staff bylaws addressing this conduct. Second, in all cases, a root cause analysis should be performed to approach the situation objectively so that both parties stand to benefit. This step will avoid the appearance of any economic impropriety or other attendant causes of bias or favoritism. Third, this analysis should be performed under the auspices of a protected peer-review process, establishing privilege from legal discovery in most jurisdictions—although this varies state by state, with protection from legal proceedings overturned by statutory intervention. Fourth, an alternative dispute resolution process, such as mediation or nonbinding or binding arbitration, often provides a more satisfactory resolution for all parties involved than an adversarial litigation process involving judicial intervention (Table 2.2).

TABLE 2.2. Medical staff quality-of-care conflict approach [4].

1. Familiarization with provisions regarding questioning of care quality
2. Root cause analytic approach
3. Peer-review protection for analysis
4. Mediation rather than litigation

References

1. Veltman L. The disruptive physician: the risk manager's role. J Healthc Risk Manag. 1995;15(2):11–6.
2. Haun JP. A process for objective review of physician performance. Physician Exec. 1992;18(3):51–5.
3. Martin WF. Is your hospital safe? Disruptive behavior and workplace bullying. Hosp Top. 2008;86(3):21–8.
4. Zbar RI, Taylor LD, Canady JW. The disruptive physician: righteous maverick or dangerous pariah. Plastic Reconstruct Surg. 2009;123(1):409–15.

Chapter 3
Organizational Approach

The complex issue of disruptive behavior by health-care professionals has been addressed by many formal medical organizations, including specialty associations, state licensing boards, medical societies, and consultant and regulatory oversight groups. Based on its 2000 report, the American Medical Association (AMA) [1] issued Opinion 9.045—Physicians with Disruptive Behavior—as part of its code of ethics. This formal opinion, however, covers only the conduct of individual physicians and does not address the collective behavior of the other health-care providers in the system, which is covered separately.

First, the AMA describes *disruptive behavior* as "personal conduct," whether verbal or physical, that affects or potentially may affect patient care, including actions that interfere with one's ability to work with other members of the health-care team. This definition specifically excludes good faith criticism or suggestions offered in an attempt to improve patient care. Second, the AMA recommends that each medical staff adopt bylaws and provisions for intervention, provide procedural safeguards to protect due process, and offer professional wellness opportunities to assist the people involved. Third, it suggests that several elements be addressed during development of the disruptive behavior policy, specifically in the document and working plan (Table 3.1) [1].

© Springer International Publishing Switzerland 2016
R.B. Vukmir, *Disruptive Healthcare Provider Behavior*,
DOI 10.1007/978-3-319-27924-4_3

TABLE 3.1. Physicians with disruptive behavior (AMA Opinion 9.045) [1].

1. Personal conduct, verbal, or physical that may cause actual or potential negative outcomes in patient care constitute disruptive behavior
2. Medical staff should adopt bylaws, due process protections, and wellness alternatives
3. Policy development should include identified specific elements in the protocol

First, the policy should include a clear statement of principal objectives to ensure high patient care standards and promote a professional practice and work environment (Table 3.2). Second, it should clearly define the behaviors that require intervention, rather than leaving the matter open to individualized, variable interpretation. Third, it should provide a mechanism to report, track, record, and analyze individual events and to compile this information into a working database to allow current shortcomings to be addressed and future care to be improved. Fourth, the policy should provide a process whereby reports of disruptive behavior can be independently verified and corroborated, ideally by a party with no competitive or financial interest that might give the appearance of bias. Fifth, it should establish a tracking process whereby a physician is notified, in a timely fashion, that a report has been filed, allowing adequate time for him or her to respond. Sixth, the policy also should allow for a monitoring program to track potential improvement after intervention, and this program should offer a corrective pathway for improvement.

Seventh, the policy should ensure that the corrective action is commensurate with the severity of the issue that has been factually substantiated. It is important to avoid overreacting to the behavior in question. The path chosen most often, seeking suspension or discharge of the provider, should be the last resort, after self-corrective or structured

TABLE 3.2. Elements of a disruptive behavior policy [1].

1. Clearly stated objectives to ensure high-quality patient care standards and a professional practice environment
2. Description of the behavior types that require intervention
3. A mechanism to report and record
4. A process to review and verify reports
5. Notification system to report and to provide an opportunity to respond
6. A monitoring system to track intervention
7. A means to ensure that corrective action is commensurate with the focus issue
8. Identification of the individuals involved in the process: analysis and monitoring
9. Explicit guidelines to protect the identity of the reporter

rehabilitative approaches have been taken. On the other hand, disruptive behavior should not be ignored or dismissed and must be dealt with decisively in a protocolized fashion. Eighth, the policy should stress the importance of identifying the individuals involved in all steps of the evaluation process: reporting, reviewing, analyzing, and monitoring. Again, the goal is to determine and track the process of remediation, which is the desired end point. Ninth, it is crucial that the policy provides a reporting pathway that protects the confidentiality of reporting individuals, which is especially important when the reporter has a role classified at a different level of the command hierarchy. Typical examples include a paraprofessional provider reporting a nurse, a nurse reporting a physician, and a physician reporting an administrator.

Clearly, the most effective approach to managing disruptive behavior involves definitive guidelines offered by high-integrity, external professional agencies such as the AMA. Likewise, in July 2008, the Joint Commission issued a Sentinel Event Alert titled Behaviors That Undermine a Culture of Safety [2]. Then on January 1, 2009, it established a new Leadership Standard, LD.03.01.01, which addresses disruptive behavior in three distinct areas [3]. First, the Joint Commission defined the elements of performance to include EP.4, which states that the facility has a code of conduct that defines both acceptable and unacceptable or disruptive behaviors. Second, it memorialized EP.5, in which facility leaders develop and implement a process to manage disruptive behaviors. Third, in the medical staff standards (MS.4), the commission added interpersonal skills and professionalism to the six core competencies required for the credentialing process.

The Joint Commission also recommended activities to ensure a successful intervention program for disruptive behavior (Table 3.3). First, all team members—physicians and nonphysician health-care providers—should be educated

TABLE 3.3. Joint Commission disruptive behavior program [3].

1. Educate all team members on the appropriate code of conduct
2. Hold all team members accountable and enforce the code consistently
3. Include these essential policy and procedure tenets
   a. "Zero tolerance" for disruptive behavior
   b. Complementary physician and nonphysician programs
   c. Clear reporter protections
   d. Involvement of patients and families in resolution
   e. Definition of disciplinary action triggers
4. Use a multidisciplinary interventional team
5. Provide skill-based training to all leaders and team members
6. Assess staff perceptions of the behavior–patient care interface
7. Develop a surveillance and reporting system involving ombudsman to assess patient and family affect
8. Support the surveillance system with a tiered, supportive, patient-focused program
9. Focus on staff well-being and have adequate resources for the task
10. Encourage interprofessional dialogue using different communication forums
11. Document all issues and interventions

on appropriate behavior defined in a code of conduct. Programs ensuring that all staff members are informed and knowledgeable are the most successful. Second, all team members should be accountable and should enforce the code consistently among staff members. Nothing scuttles a program faster than the appearance of favoritism in the evaluation or implementation process.

Third, policies and procedures that specify crucial tenets of performance should be developed and implemented. These guidelines should include a "zero-tolerance" policy for disruptive behavior; complementary, parallel programs for physicians and nonphysicians; demonstrable reporter protections; involvement of patients or families; and a definition of disciplinary action triggers. These triggers may include suspension, loss of privileges, termination, or reports to the appropriate medical licensing body. Whereas some triggers are automatic and require external reporting immediately, others allow more time for consideration and remediation before an external report must be filed.

Fourth, to take the most effective approach, a multidisciplinary team should be developed that involves physicians, nurses, auxiliary providers, administrators, and other employees to address these behaviors. A true 360-degree evaluation program targeting the upper administrative chain of command is useful. Fifth, all leaders and team members should be given skill-based training emphasizing team building and collaborative practice. Providers are more likely to be successful if they feel they have a voice in the overall operation. Sixth, a program should be developed to monitor the staff's perception of the undesirable behavior–patient care interface for adverse trends. Members should be solicited regarding their opinions on what approaches or strategies will and will not work in a particular environment or patient care scenario.

Seventh, a surveillance and reporting system, possibly anonymous, should be established for ombudsman and advocacy services to note patient and family concerns. However, the person overseeing this system ideally should have experience in patient care, as this is difficult territory to navigate correctly. Eighth, the surveillance program should be supported with tiered, nonconfrontational strategies to provide corrective action in a stepwise fashion. This program should be nonadversarial, beginning with an informal approach with a planned structure centered on trust and accountability for all while remaining focused on patient safety as the definitive end point.

Ninth, all interventions should be carried out with staff well-being as the central focus, with adequate resources to complete the task. Tenth, interprofessional dialogue should be encouraged across several different communication modes to encourage participation by all parties. Some people interact more productively by email, others by voice, or by face to face; therefore, the communication style should be chosen based on what works best for the parties involved. Eleventh, all data regarding surveys, analysis, and interventions directed toward eliminating institutional disruptive behavior should be documented. This documentation may include comments viewed as unfavorable to the system or administration; however, it is essential that they be included both for face validity and to improve the process itself.

In November 2011, the Joint Commission redefined the term *disruptive behavior* based on several influencing factors, with the behavior being the final common pathway [4]. Some physicians felt that the term is ambiguous and might be misinterpreted, especially in situations in which a particular provider is a strong advocate of improved patient care. Therefore, the commission instituted the more descriptive term *behavior that undermines a culture of safety* and incorporated it into 2012 accreditation manuals.

The Joint Commission then began requiring health-care organizations to support a program to investigate and help resolve disruptive behavior in the workplace. Stecker et al. [5] surveyed 617 participants by questionnaire and found that disruptive behavior is pervasive. This type of conduct was noted by 82 % of the organizations studied, with 74 % of staff members stating that they witnessed this behavior and 5 %

reporting that they personally experienced it. It is clear, then, that disruptive behavior is encountered in a significant proportion of cases.

Most importantly, all health-care organizations not only are encouraged, but now are required at the leadership level to enact standards to address disruptive behavior. In conclusion, it is clear that disruptive behavior in the health-care arena may involve any member of the team and is addressed most effectively via a cooperative approach focusing on staff wellness, quality of care, and patient safety.

References

1. AMA. AMA Code of medical ethics. Opinion 9.045-physicians with disruptive behavior. December 2000. http://www.ama-assn.org/ama/pub/physician-resources/medical-ethics/code-medical-ethics/opinion9045.page. Accessed 4 March 2012.
2. The Joint Commission. Sentinel event alert: behaviors that undermine a culture of safety. Issue 40, July 9, 2008. www.jointcommission.org/SentinelEvents/SentinelEventAlert/sea_40.htm. Accessed 20 Sept 2010.
3. Joint Commission Perspectives. Revision to LD.03.01.01, EPs 4 and 5. Jt Comm Accred Healthcare Organ. 2012;32(1):7.
4. The Joint Commission. The term "Disruptive Behavior" is changed as it applies to physicians. Nov 29, 2011. https://www.andersonservices.com/blog/2011/11/jcaho-changes-the-term-disruptive-behavior-as-it-relatestophysicans/. Accessed 4 Mar 2012.
5. Stecker M, Epstein N, Stecker MM. Analysis of inter-provider conflicts among healthcare providers. Surg Neurol Int. 2013;4 Suppl 5:S375–82.

Chapter 4
Maturation of the Analysis

An interesting trend has developed over time concerning analysis of the disruptive behavior conundrum (Table 4.1). Historically, the issue raised tended to focus on a single person or behavior rather than on an interface between a system and multiple participants in the event. It was felt that this behavior was a problem resting solely with the physician, and therefore the *disruptive physician* label was applied. It became recognized, however, that perhaps it was not the individual who was undesirable but rather the behavior itself, and so the use of the descriptor *disruptive physician behavior* replaced the *disruptive physician* label.

Later, a question arose regarding whether it is the individual or the system that is the culprit. Earlier, more rudimentary analysis suggested that the problem lies in a few "bad" individuals working in a "good" system, which clearly is folly. As our analysis matured and became more insightful, we recognized that the issues that arise often are more complex and that indeed systemic issues often are the drivers of the controversy. Therefore, the solution often requires improvement of the overall system as well as modification of an individual's behavior.

This issue was raised by Leape et al. [1], who suggested a system-level solution to "problem doctors," postulating that individual provider failures are exacerbated by system stressors. According to these authors, the proper approach is a four-stage model that focuses on adopting standards, requiring compliance, monitoring performance, and responding to the deficiencies found (Table 4.2).

© Springer International Publishing Switzerland 2016   17
R.B. Vukmir, *Disruptive Healthcare Provider Behavior*,
DOI 10.1007/978-3-319-27924-4_4

TABLE 4.1. Difficult encounter matrix.

1. Is it the person or the behavior that is disruptive?
2. Is the individual or the system at fault?
3. Are both physicians and nurses involved?
4. Is it a patient care not a staff issue?
5. Is the label being used inappropriately?
6. Are the issues related to patients as well as providers?

TABLE 4.2. Four-stage model to address disruptive behavior [1].

1. Adopt standards
2. Require compliance
3. Monitor performance
4. Respond to deficiencies

It later became apparent that disruptive behavior is not just a physician problem; other providers, including nurses, administrators, and other health-care professionals, also exhibit this conduct. Interestingly, this behavior has been observed among nonphysician providers as often as among physician providers.

Rosenstein and O'Daniel [2, 3] performed and subsequently refined their study of 102 VHA hospitals in which 4530 respondents, including 2846 nurses, 944 physicians, and 40 administrators completed a questionnaire concerning disruptive behavior. Among the staff members who responded, 77 % — including 88 % of the nurses and 51 % of the physicians — stated that they had witnessed disruptive behavior in physicians. The more interesting aspect, however, is that 65 % of the respondents — 73 % of the nurses and 48 % of the physicians — also witnessed disruptive behavior committed by the nurses at their facility. Furthermore, 67 % of the respondents thought disruptive behaviors were associated with adverse patient care events in the health-care arena. They specifically cited staff dissatisfaction (75 %), detrimental quality effects (72 %), medical errors (71 %), adverse events (66 %), and patient safety concerns (53 %) occurring in this group. Twenty-five percent of the respondents believed that disruptive conduct resulted in patient mortality (Table 4.3). Based on these observations, the authors made several recommendations, including preventing disruptive events from occurring in the first place, responding in "real time" to prevent harm to staff harm, and initiating a postreview action and follow-up plan to sustain improvement.

The next phase of analysis maturation veered from predominantly provider-centric issues to patient safety concerns. Rather than being centered on a nexus of staff conflict, the focus began to shift toward the actual or potential adverse impact on patient safety as well as creation of a plan to mitigate this effect. Clearly, most hospital dilemmas today are analyzed based on the patient care perspective rather than focusing on staff alone.

More recently, a critical change occurred regarding the label *disruptive physician* when it was acknowledged that this pejorative term has been used inappropriately to describe physicians who speak out about patient care issues in good faith. In these cases, the touchstone used to define "proper behavior" is that it occurred before the provider was labeled disruptive, normal quality reporting channels were used, and proper procedures for analysis were followed. However, if the provider invoked a patient care issue after the fact, using inappropriate reporting channels and dialogue, the behavior more likely was self-serving, and the disruptive classification is appropriate (Table 4.4).

TABLE 4.3. Disruptive behavior association [2, 3].

Effect of behavior	Respondents reporting (%)
Staff dissatisfaction	75
Detrimental quality effects	72
Medical errors	71
Adverse events	66
Patient safety compromise	53
Patient mortality	25

TABLE 4.4. Appropriateness of the behavior.

Behavior	Appropriate	Inappropriate
Timing	Before label	After label
Process	Standard reporting	Alternative reporting
Focus	Patient	Provider

Reynolds [4] cited a 3–5 % incidence of physicians who alleged to have engaged in disruptive behavior in the health-care setting. In his recent treatise, however, he suggests that "the disruptive label should not be applied to physicians just because they present controversial ideas or offer criticism of the established medical system." Likewise, "a single episode of disruptive behavior does not render one a 'disruptive physician.' Human beings are complex creatures, no one is perfect, and expecting absolute harmony in any workplace is unrealistic" [4]. However, every conceivable effort must be made to ensure harmonious interactions in the health-care arena so that patient care is not adversely affected.

Perhaps, then, the most accurate way to describe these events is in terms of a *difficult encounter* rather than a *difficult provider*. In this way, the problem is ascribed to a particular interaction among multiple individuals or parties. Likewise, many environmental or situational factors can influence the outcome of any health-care event. Most experts have come to realize that patients and their families, as well as other outside elements, may have an equal role in driving some of these events. In fact, corollary publications have been written about the "difficult patient" or "difficult encounter" that has been directed toward the patient and the provider in equal measure.

Therefore, a difficult encounter is the compilation of effects from a diverse matrix of interactions among physicians, patients, and situational factors [5]. Physician factors that have been described include a negative bias toward particular disease conditions, poor communication skills, managerial or administrative challenges, and situational stressors. Patient factors that have been implicated include personality disorders, drug or alcohol abuse, multiple poorly defined disease symptoms, medical noncompliance, and self-destructive behavior. Situational factors that may compound problems for both patients and providers include time pressures, patient or staff conflicts, and complex social issues (Table 4.5).

A physician can manage a difficult encounter successfully by following a defined formulaic approach that emphasizes the use of empathetic listening skills to achieve the end point set by a goal-sharing team and taking a nonjudgmental, caring attitude and approach in his or her interactions with all providers involved. An effective comprehensive evaluation should be performed to determine whether medical and/or psychological disorders played a role in the event. Often, monitoring the impact of present or past physical or psychological abuse may be an enlightening tool for facilitating understanding of current events.

The most effective plans for managing difficult patient encounters include the delineation and enforcement of reasonable operational boundaries, as well as the use of focused patient-centered communication. Moreover, as with any other negotiation process, a mutually agreed upon care plan

TABLE 4.5. The difficult encounter matrix [5].

A. Physician factors
  1. Disease-specific bias
  2. Poor communication skills
  3. Situational stressors
B. Patient factors
  1. Personality disorders
  2. Multiple poorly defined disease symptoms
  3. Medical noncompliance
  4. Self-destructive behavior
C. Situational factors
  1. Time pressures
  2. Patient and staff conflicts
  3. Complex social issues

TABLE 4.6. Management of the difficult encounter [5].

1. Use empathetic listening skills
2. Take a nonjudgmental, caring attitude
3. Consider underlying medical or psychiatric disease
4. Consider past or present physical or mental abuse
5. Set reasonable boundaries
6. Use patient-centered communication
7. Mutually agree on a treatment plan

will lead to a more productive outcome than a unilaterally imposed one (Table 4.6). In conclusion, the ability to successfully navigate a difficult encounter rests with understanding, setting expectations, and negotiating away the less significant issues to achieve group consensus.

References

1. Leape LL, Fromson JA. Problem doctors: is there a system-level solution? Ann Intern Med. 2006;144(2):107–15.
2. Rosenstein AH, O'Daniel M. Managing disruptive physician behavior: impact on staff relationships and patient care. Neurology. 2008;70(17):1564–70.
3. Rosenstein AH, O'Daniel M. A survey of the impact of disruptive behaviors and communication defects on patient safety. Jt Comm J Qual Patient Saf. 2008;34(8):464–71.
4. Reynolds NT. Disruptive physician behavior: use and misuse of the label. J Med Regul. 2012;98(1):8–19.
5. Cannarella LR, Jacques CH, Donovan C, Cottrell S, Buck J. Managing difficult encounters: understanding physician, patient and situational factors. Am Fam Physician. 2013;87(6):419–25.

Chapter 5
Profile of the Behavior

Clearly, effective analysis, intervention, and improvement begin after identifying the situational attributes that make problem-prone behavior even more likely to occur in the often stressful health-care setting.

The scope of the problem was defined in 1994 by a British National Health Service (NHS) study sample collected during a 5-year period in a large health-care setting [1]. The NHS found that 6 % of its senior staff physicians (49 of 850) exhibited behaviors resulting in a disciplinary inquiry. The problems encountered included working with a poor attitude, disruptive or irresponsible behavior (33 %), lack of commitment to duties (22 %), poor skills or inadequate knowledge (20 %), dishonesty (11 %), sexual matters (7 %), disorganized practice and poor communication (5 %), and other reported findings (2 %). After disciplinary proceedings, more than half of these providers (51 %) left their facility, whereas 43 % continued working at the site after counseling or supervisory intervention. This study, however, has several limitations, with some critics arguing that the parameters used for analysis at the time were too rudimentary to be effective. Moreover, the survey questions focused more on competence than on behavioral anomalies or aberrant interactions in the workplace. In addition, local and regional variations exist with regard to behaviors that rise to the level of being called "disruptive." Therefore, the identification of problem-prone behavior requires standardized terminology and analysis to be most accurate.

© Springer International Publishing Switzerland 2016
R.B. Vukmir, *Disruptive Healthcare Provider Behavior*,
DOI 10.1007/978-3-319-27924-4_5

For any disruptive behavior program to be truly effective, its monitoring, tracking, and interventional functions should be directed at the problem behavior rather than at the individual, although this path often is more difficult.

The American Congress of Obstetricians and Gynecologists (ACOG) Committee on Patient Safety and Quality Improvement described disruptive behavior as "interaction that can create distress or negatively affect morale in the workplace" [2]. The committee offered specific examples of this behavior, citing yelling, insulting, or refusal to perform his or her duties as the most common types of issues encountered (Table 5.1). Its findings also include overt verbal, physical, or sexual boundary violations, as well as more subtle nonverbal gestures or passive–aggressive behavior. The ACOG committee found that these events typically occurred among only a minority of physicians (3–5 %) and usually were targeted at a coworker in a lower-level position in the workplace hierarchy [2, 3], such as auxiliary personnel, nurses, medical students, or resident physicians.

The Medical Council of New Zealand [4] published its own list of behaviors that deems unprofessional and likely to have an adverse impact on the health-care team and patient safety (Table 5.2). Most of the items on the list are blatant and would be obvious to the observer, including intimidation; sexual harassment; ethnic slurs; loud, abusive comments; and threats of violence, retribution, or litigation. Again, however, significant regional and geographic variations exist in the behaviors described.

TABLE 5.1. Examples of disruptive behavior cited by ACOG [2].

1. Using profane or disrespectful language
2. Yelling, berating, or insulting coworkers
3. Throwing instruments, charts, or other objects
4. Bullying, demeaning, or intimidating dialogue
5. Criticizing providers or organizations to patients in front of staff
6. Making overt or suggestive sexual comments
7. Use of sarcasm, nonverbal gestures, or passive–aggressive behavior

TABLE 5.2. Unprofessional behavior and the health-care team [4].

1. Intimidation or bullying tactics
2. Sexual harassment
3. Racial, ethnic, or sexist comments
4. Loud, rude comments
5. Abusive, profane, or offensive language
6. Systematic, persistent tardiness in responding to requests
7. Throwing instruments or charts
8. Offensive sarcasm
9. Threats of violence, retribution, or vexatious litigation
10. Demands for exclusive treatment
11. Passive–aggressive behaviors
12. Disrespect to dependent personnel in care transition

With regard to identifying problem behavior, increased attention has been paid to less noticeable, more subtle interactions that may have an equally intimidating effect. Although the days of screaming, throwing charts, destroying property, and storming out of care settings should be long past, less obvious behaviors exist that should be noted as well. These actions include persistent lateness and failure to respond to a patient's request for discussion or consultation or to questions concerning an order entry or other patient management inquiry. A typical example is a provider who typically responds only after the second or third page, the rationale being "if it's important they'll call back."

Other examples of more subtle but problematic conduct are demands for special treatment regarding particular office accommodations, decorating requests, operating room design, and selection of personnel or protocols used for the provider's patients or circumstances. In the highly competitive hospital environment, once one provider's requests are accommodated, demands from other providers often follow.

Another example is the so-called passive–aggressive behavior, whereby a provider may appear to be agreeable in public but, behind the scenes, is negative and resistant to change even though his or her external behavior is socially acceptable. He or she may request additional meetings, consultation, and analysis of the plan under discussion, beyond the usual level of inquiry. When the team reaches a consensus and solutions are offered, the provider objects to the plan's implementation and to any change beyond the status quo. This type of behavior also may be observed in a provider at the care transition point or interface, when he or she is unwilling to discuss care issues with colleagues and personnel, although they are being supervised in a cordial manner.

A closer look at the passive–aggressive behavior continuum allows a better understanding of the disruptive provider profile (Table 5.3) [5]. Again, these are more subtle behaviors, such as hostile avoidance of dialogue, the proverbial "cold shoulder," speaking in a quiet or muffled voice, or intentionally miscommunicating important information to others in the health-care team and then being promoted to a higher position in the institution when he or she discovers and corrects the error. The theatrical display then becomes an integral part of the care process, providing ongoing distraction.

Obviously, concerns also exist when the passive–aggressive conduct is more blatant. More overt behaviors include condescending language or tone, excessive sarcasm, sexual innuendo, malicious gossip or inappropriate humor, and jokes about a person's appearance (Table 5.4). Also important are

TABLE 5.3. Passive–aggressive behaviors [5].

1. Hostile avoidance—the "cold shoulder"
2. Intentional miscommunication
3. Unresponsiveness to professional requests—paging or consultation
4. Speaking in an inaudible volume
5. Condescending language and tone
6. Impatience with questions or with having to educate
7. Participating in malicious gossip
8. "Joking" about race, gender, sexual orientation, or religion
9. Commenting on personal appearance
10. Implied threats of retribution for filing a complaint

TABLE 5.4. Overt disruptive behavior [5].

1. Condescending language or tone
2. Excessive sarcasm
3. Sexual innuendo
4. Malicious gossip
5. Inappropriate jokes
6. Personal humor

the method and style of communication; for example, impatience with questions, explanations, and education of other staff is problematic in the health-care arena.

As noted earlier, one of the most pervasive problematic behaviors encountered in many facilities is a physician being unavailable when summoned for professional matters while on call. This may be systemic problem in which the provider repeatedly ignores pages until the second or third call, berates the person who requests aid, and/or delays consultation and evaluation. Monitoring of the aforementioned subtle behaviors, therefore, is critically important to establish trends and establish patterns for improvement.

Goettler et al. [6] performed a retrospective blinded study at a 751-bed hospital employing 640 physicians on its active staff roster. They reported that overall, 18 % of the physicians (114) had been involved in disruptive behavior event, whereas 7 % (44) were the subject of multiple reports. The latter group accounted for most (63 %) of the reports filed, with 61 % of these practitioners (27) being reported twice, 18 % three times, 9 % four times, and 7 % five times; one physician was reported to have been involved in disruptive behavior events (Table 5.5). Although the multiple-report group had more communication issues cited than the single-report cohort; however, no significant differences were noted in patient outcome.

The authors found an association between specialty group and disruptive behavior, with anesthesiology, cardiology, hospitalists, orthopedics, trauma, and obstetrics/gynecology having a higher incidence of this behavior than other medical practitioners in the study sample (Table 5.6). They also observed a difference between genders, with female physicians

TABLE 5.5. Group with multiple reports of disruptive behavior in Goettler et al. [6] study[a].

Events reported (*n*)	Multiple-report physicians (%)
2	61
3	18
4	9
5	7
6	1

[a]The multiple-report group was responsible for 63 % of all events reported

TABLE 5.6. Specialties with the highest incidence of disruptive behavior [6].

1. Anesthesia
2. Cardiology
3. Hospitalist
4. Orthopedics
5. Trauma
6. Obstetrics/gynecology

less likely than males to be reported in a disruptive behavior incident. Interestingly, reports filed by nonphysician staff were more likely to be directed against physicians in the same clinical practice area (80 %; 74 of 94 cases). However, most reports filed by physicians (72 %, 18 of 25) involved those outside their clinical practice area. This is an interesting phenomenon in which reporting incidence was affected by both job role and service line. As an example, nurses tended to file reports against physicians they worked with in their own service area, whereas physicians tended not to file reports on those in their own service line; their reports targeted staff outside their working group. The authors, however, simply commented on their observations without offering theories on causality or significance.

Although quality improvement organizations must strive to make these incidents "never" events, it must be recognized that fewer than 1 % of these reports are found to be valid or definably disruptive to the health-care delivery process. The overwhelming majority of these events (99 %) in fact were not disruptive if analyzed based on clearly defined guidelines with patient care as the outcome variable. Therefore, to obtain the most useful information, standardized, objective peer review using explicit criteria is an essential part of the analysis of events such as these. Although it is important to recognize that a defined change in outcome often is difficult to prove, that does not mean that disruptive behavior does not result in patient harms that are more difficult to measure. The patient safety interface often is invoked as a defense or explanatory rationale in discussions regarding a dysfunctional culture.

Leape et al. [7] classified disrespectful behavior in the health-care setting into six categories (Table 5.7): (1) disruptive behavior (which the authors define and for which they give examples); (2) demeaning treatment of nurses, residents, and students; (3) passive–aggressive behavior; (4) passive disrespect; (5) dismissive treatment of patients; and (6) systemic disrespect. The authors posited that disrespectful behavior may be partly rooted in the physician's own insecurity but sometimes is tolerated by a hierarchical hospital system and exacerbated by increased production pressure. Every physician has a complex, multifaceted mix of positive and negative attributes that may vary over time depending on circumstances. Therefore, although general trends may be extrapolated, individual site-based solutions often are required.

On the positive side, physicians typically are intelligent, highly skilled, hard-working, confident, and persevering

TABLE 5.7. Types of disrespectful behavior reported by Leape et al. [7].

1. Disruptive behavior
2. Demeaning treatment of nurses, residents, or students
3. Passive–aggressive behavior
4. Passive disrespect
5. Dismissive treatment of patients
6. Systemic disrespect

members of the health-care team (Table 5.8) [5]. However, some may possess more problematic traits, including arrogance; controlling, inflexible behaviors; exaggerated self-importance; a tendency to deny or project blame onto others; vindictiveness; and litigiousness [5]. Obviously, this is an overly simplistic analysis, but it helps define a conceptual rather than a specific understanding of such a complex issue.

As noted earlier, the focus often is on the individual rather on a more systematic, multifactorial problem. Senior-level, experienced administrators should recognize that on closer inspection, almost invariably, a true medical care issue lies at the core of the controversy. Often the method available for raising a complaint is flawed; therefore, reporting systems must be improved to obtain the most accurate information for analysis. Fundamental fairness requires that if an individual behavior is cited, a specialty-matched, peer-review evaluation should be undertaken by a clinically active physician to provide the most effective remediation and improvement plan.

Just as important as knowing what a disruptive behavior "is," it is equally vital to know what disruptive behavior "is not." Every health-care provider or administrator may have a bad day under a particular set of circumstances and react in negative ways. However, his or her behavior achieves significance only when a pattern of disruptive behavior develops that is repetitive, consistent, or egregious. This is the

TABLE 5.8. Physician skill set balance [5].

Positive	Negative
Intelligent	Arrogant
Highly skilled	Controlling
Hard working	Inflexible
Confident	Self-important
Persevering	Tendency to deny
Cooperative	Tendency to project
Loyal	Vindictive
Dedicated	Litigious

point at which intervention should begin with monitoring, analysis, and tracking to minimize the effects of the disruptive behavior and to ensure a positive health-care experience for patients.

References

1. Donaldson LJ. Doctors with problems in an NHS workforce. BMJ. 1994;308(6939):1277–82.
2. American College of Obstetricians and Gynecologists— Committee Opinion. Disruptive behavior. Number 508, October 2011. Accessed 4 March 2012. http://www.acog.org/Resources_ And_Publications/Committee_Opinions/Committee_on_Pa
3. Leape LL, Fromson JA. Problem doctors: is there a system-level solution? Ann Intern Med. 2006;144(2):107–15.
4. Medical Council of New Zealand. Unprofessional behaviour and the health care team. Protecting patient safety. August 2009.
5. Reynolds NT. Disruptive physician behavior: use and misuse of the label. J Med Regul. 2012;98(1):8–19.
6. Goettler CE, Butler TS, Shackleford P, Rotondo MF. Physician behavior: not ready for 'never' land. Am Surg. 2011;77(12): 1600–5.
7. Leape LL, Shore MF, Dienstag JL, Mayer RJ, Edgman-Levitan S, Meyer GS, Healy GB. Perspective: a culture of respect, Part 1: The nature and causes of disrespectful behavior by physicians. Acad Med. 2012;87(7):845–52.

Chapter 6
Location at Risk

Many opinions exist concerning the hospital locations and service lines most at risk for disruptive behavior, with several areas figuring prominently in studies and analyses of this issue.

6.1 Operating Suite

Using a questionnaire-based survey, Rosenstein and O'Daniel [1] compared the reporting of disruptive behavior in the perioperative area of a large academic medical center with a national database and found that disruptive behaviors are significantly more common in the operating suite than other hospital areas. In addition, they found that most times, the attending surgeon was the individual exhibiting the disruptive conduct [1]. The authors suggested that this type of behavior may increase stress, impair concentration, and hinder communication, relationships, and collaboration among health-care providers. To address this problem, they recommend an institution-level commitment to awareness, recognition, education, policy, and adherence to procedures.

Not surprisingly, perceptions vary with regard to what constitutes intimidation in the health-care setting depending on one's perspective of the controversy. A survey of physicians in the perioperative arena revealed that a majority agreed that behaviors identified as intimidating by national organizations actually constituted intimidation in only four of nine cases (44.4 %) [2]. This disparity between the physician group

© Springer International Publishing Switzerland 2016
R.B. Vukmir, *Disruptive Healthcare Provider Behavior*,
DOI 10.1007/978-3-319-27924-4_6

and the organizations was found in even the most egregious examples of disruptive behavior.

Therefore, arriving at a consensus regarding solutions is difficult when there is so much disagreement over the barometer of measurement or entry into the process itself. Often, a focused program is needed to educate the operating room staff on how to identify and acknowledge the problem as well as to work together to arrive at a solution.

6.2   Labor and Delivery

Another area of concern is the labor and delivery area, where a disproportionate number of reports of disruptive behavior have been cited. Veltman [3] conducted a questionnaire-based survey of nurse managers in West Coast obstetrics units and found a 60.7 % rate of disruptive behavior exhibited by a wide range of professionals [3]. He concluded that these incidents contributed to near misses in patient care, adverse events, and excessive turnover in nursing staff and that traditional approaches to addressing these behaviors are discouraged, are often ineffective, and require newer and better interventions to ensure a safe patient care environment. It should be noted, however, that this sample was solicited from a group of unified system nurse managers, which should be taken into consideration when interpreting the results more widely.

6.3   Intensive Care/Critical Care Unit

The critical care or intensive care unit (ICU) is another high-stress area often prone to disruption during normal day-to-day operations. Piquette et al. [4] conducted 32 semistructured interviews of ICU personnel and noted a precarious balance of negatives, including high workload, risk, and responsibility, although resources usually were in place to meet these demands. Disruptive behaviors often occur when a system is under stress and needed resources are not available. However, the ICU is best suited to deal with high patient acuity and emergencies; therefore, this rationale cannot be used as an excuse to justify the behavior. The first question to ask when confronted with a disruptive event in a critical care unit was whether the necessary resources and backup were available to the affected patients and providers. These incidents appear to be related to the individual provider involved and correlate with changing patient conditions, an unpredictable deterioration in status, or a lack of expected resources. The study authors recommend matching demands and resources in times of crisis to avoid these issues.

Good medical facilities typically have the foresight to establish flexible staffing plans. More often than not, these plans involve real-time nursing staffing plans to ensure bed availability, whereas physicians are required to institute rapid disposition and discharge protocols to facilitate patient flow. Ideally, a physician "gatekeeper" is available to oversee the process and to ensure the participation of all parties.

6.4   Emergency Department

The emergency department (ED) is another high-stress area where disruptive behaviors may occur. Based on a survey of 370 ED personnel, Rosenstein and Naylor [5] found that disruptive behaviors were found in all staff working in the ED. The percentage of respondents witnessing this behavior in physicians was similar to that of those observing it in nurses: 57 % and 52 %, respectively. The survey participants also felt these incidents were associated with adverse events, medical errors, patient safety compromise, poor quality, and patient mortality (Table 6.1). However, it is important to realize that these responses were subjective staff impressions and were neither proven nor disproven.

Concerns regarding the adverse impact on team dynamics, communication efficiency, information flow, and task accountability are justified, stressing the need for monitoring and intervention. Not everything in medicine must be proven; some things are inherently obvious.

TABLE 6.1. Consequences of disruptive behavior based on Rosenstein and Naylor [5] survey.

Consequence	Respondents (%)
Poor quality	35.8
Medical errors	35.4
Adverse events	32.8
Patient safety compromise	24.7
Specific adverse event	18
Patient mortality	12.3

References

1. Rosenstein AH, O'Daniel M. Impact and implications of disruptive behavior in the perioperative arena. J Am Coll Surg. 2006; 203(1):96–105.
2. Dull DL, Fox L. Perception of intimidation in a perioperative setting. Am J Med Qual. 2010;25(2):87–94.
3. Veltman LL. Disruptive behavior in obstetrics: a hidden threat to patient safety. Am J Obstet Gynecol. 2007;196(6):587.e4–5.
4. Piquette D, Reeves S, LeBlanc VR. Stressful intensive care unit medical crises: how individual responses impact on team performance. Crit Care Med. 2009;37(4):1251–5.
5. Rosenstein AH, Naylor B. Incidence and impact of physician and nurse disruptive behaviors in the emergency department. J Emerg Med. 2012;43(1):139–48.

Chapter 7
Specialty at Risk

Just as disruptive behavior is more prevalent in certain physical locations, studies also have revealed an association between this type of conduct and specialty or service line. Indeed, Rosenstein and O'Daniel [1] found that certain specialties seem to be more prone to this behavior (Table 7.1), with surgical disciplines and some medical procedural specialties more highly represented than primary care disciplines. The practitioners most commonly associated with disruptive behavior were general surgeons, who were responsible for 31 % of the cases. Next were cardiovascular surgeons (21 %), neurosurgeons (15 %), orthopedic surgeons (7 %), cardiologists (7 %), obstetrician/gynecologists (6 %), gastroenterologists (4 %), and neurologists (4 %). The remaining medical specialists represented fewer than 3 % of the cases of disruptive behavior.

7.1 General Surgery

General surgeons appear to be the physician group most commonly labeled as exhibiting "disruptive behavior." Cochran and Elder [2] analyzed a group of 19 individuals with various occupations working in the perioperative setting and used a grounded theory methodology to evaluate the impact in that environment. Among the adverse events they noted was a shift in attention from the patient to the surgeon, with all of its attendant complications. When staff members

© Springer International Publishing Switzerland 2016
R.B. Vukmir, *Disruptive Healthcare Provider Behavior*,
DOI 10.1007/978-3-319-27924-4_7

TABLE 7.1. Specialist associated with disruptive behavior.

Specialists	Cases (%)
General surgeons	31
Cardiovascular surgeons	21
Neurosurgeons	15
Orthopedic surgeons	7
Cardiologists	7
Obstetrician/gynecologists	6
Gastroenterologists	4
Neurologists	4

Data from Rosenstein and O'Daniel [1]

became aware of disruptions, the number of procedural mistakes increased. Moreover, some of the workers who witnessed these events reported an overall diminished respect for surgeons in general. Most importantly, some observers reported that because of this behavior, they were deterred from a career in surgery (Table 7.2).

Staff members surveyed also cited coping strategies they used in the face of intimidating behaviors. They reported that talking to colleagues about their experiences was especially helpful; realizing they were not alone was an important part of the management strategy. Another coping mechanism cited by many of the respondents was externalizing the behavior, which often added to the problem. Instead of internalizing the dysphoric feelings, some staff members redirected them outward as negative emotions and affect, thereby worsening the situation. Other respondents reported that they coped with problem behavior simply by avoiding the perpetrator, which sometimes resulted in increased work loss and employee absenteeism. Lastly, the word of disruptive behavior traveled quickly among the staff members surveyed, who put unofficial "early warning" systems in place to deal with the problem. Certainly, it is better to institute programs before things deteriorate to this point in the workplace, and the staff must resort to self-help measures (Table 7.3).

TABLE 7.2. Effects of disruptive behavior in
the operating room [2].

1. Attention shift from patient to surgeon
2. Increased mistakes during procedures
3. Diminished respect for surgeons
4. Deterrence from entering surgical career

TABLE 7.3. Staff's informal coping strategies
in a disruptive environment [1].

1. Talk to colleagues
2. Externalize behavior
3. Avoid perpetrators
4. Warn other providers

Interestingly, in an earlier analysis of the same data, the same researchers expanded on the thoughts and observations of the study participants. Again, Cochran and Elder [3] described the episodes of disruptive surgeon behavior, the personality traits associated with the behavior, the environmental conditions of power, and the situations in which the behavior is demonstrated. To establish a better understanding of the disruptive behavior issue as it applies to the surgeon's thought process, they offered a series of observations.

First, they noted that the most common overt behaviors include verbal outbursts and throwing or hitting objects. Second, they postulated that the surgical training process itself either creates or attracts people of a particular personality type who may be predisposed to the behavior. Third, they suggested that the surgical arena often is the epicenter of this phenomenon because of the presence of unchecked power, significant financial productivity for the institution, and a strong hierarchical culture with subordinate personnel. Fourth, they found the most frequent situational stressor is a poor or unanticipated outcome of the surgical procedure. Fifth, they cited the presence of unfamiliar team members as a factor that often exacerbates the situation (Tables 7.4 and 7.5).

The key to handling these and other complex dilemmas in the medical setting is a successful team-building approach.

TABLE 7.4. Disruptive behavior in the general surgical arena [3].

1. Overt physical outbursts and behaviors
2. Surgical training and personality interface
3. Predisposing factors
4. Poor or unanticipated outcome
5. Unfamiliar team members

TABLE 7.5. Predisposing factors in the surgical arena [3].

1. Unchecked power
2. Financial productivity
3. Strong hierarchical tradition
4. Subordinate personnel

Sax [4] described a program to build high-performance teams in the operating room setting that includes the following components: First, the program must have clearly delineated goals to be successful. Second, each team member must understand his or her contribution to achieving the overall goal. Third, continuous feedback is necessary to facilitate team goals. Fourth, each staff member's perspective must shift from a solo to a team mentality to encourage success. Fifth, strong administrative input and support is needed to increase staff buy-in and ensure the overall success of the program (Table 7.6). This conceptual model facilitates understanding of the prevalence of the behavior as well as the resulting negative effects from the manipulation of staff and trainees, allowing both personnel and management to broker the strengths of the current program to improve the surgical environment.

7.2   Obstetrics/Gynecology

Concerns regarding disruptive behavior often focus on the obstetrics/gynecology service line because obstetric care often is given over a prolonged time continuum, with multiple

TABLE 7.6. Requirements for building a high-performance surgical team [4].

1. Delineation of clear goals
2. Each team member's understanding of his or her contribution
3. Continuous feedback
4. Team mentality
5. Strong administrative support

TABLE 7.7. Approach to addressing location- or service line-specific behaviors [5].

1. Stress placed on positive approaches
2. Mutual understanding
3. Shared goals and priorities
4. Adherence to accepted standards of care

personnel delivering vital care in the complete progression from labor to delivery [5]. High-stress, high-risk situations such as these are best addressed with a comprehensive multidisciplinary approach involving all providers in the process. Interventions should occur prospectively with the education and empowerment of all personnel to confront disruptive behavior. Once the behavior is identified, it should be addressed by a program fully supported by the administration to correct the problem.

A protocol stressing positive approaches, mutual understanding, shared goals and priorities, and adherence to accepted standards of care will improve both staff communication and patient care outcome (Table 7.7). A successful program has strong organizational commitment, has leadership support to encourage provider awareness, and includes policies, procedures, and curricula to educate and train personnel to recognize a disruptive situation (Table 7.8).

Lyndon et al. [6] used a scenario-based measure to estimate clinicians' assessment of potential harm and their likelihood of speaking up about it. The likelihood of a physician or

TABLE 7.8. Attributes of a successful behavioral management system [6].

1. Strong organizational commitment
2. Leadership support
3. Programs to improve provider awareness
4. Implementation of policies and procedures
5. Education and training programs
6. Improvement of situational awareness

TABLE 7.9. Likelihood of reporting disruptive behavior [6].

1. Likelihood is greater with higher perception of harm or injury
2. Likelihood is correlated with greater experience
3. Physicians are less likely to perceive harm
4. Nurses seem more likely to report

nurse speaking out was correlated with a greater perception of patient harm, his or her role in the care process, his or her experience in the specialty (13.7 ± 11 years on average), and the location of service delivery. Physicians often rated potential harm lower than nurses on a scale of 2 to 10 (7.5 vs. 8.4, $P < 0.001$), whereas some (12 %) indicated they were reticent to speak up regardless of the scenario. The authors suggested that the discrepancy in the severity of harm reporting may account for the differences between physicians and nurses in these study results.

The noteworthy findings and trends of this study may be summarized as follows: (1) The perception of patient harm was the biggest driver and overrode all other correlates in the study. (2) Clinicians with greater experience were more likely to cite this disruptive behavior as being aberrant in the health-care system. (3) Physicians appeared less likely to report on other providers based on perception of patient harm. (4) Nurses seemed more likely to report, probably based on a composite of the aforementioned factors (Table 7.9).

7.3   Orthopedic Surgery

Another area in which disruptive behavior is reported to be more prevalent is orthopedic surgery. Explanations offered include the high patient volume, decreased reimbursement, increased malpractice litigation, greater stress, and job dissatisfaction encountered in this specialty [7]. However, the astute commentator would recognize that these factors likely are present in all the branches of medicine and surgery practiced today (Table 7.10).

As the population ages, the orthopedic surgeon will assume an even more important role, as more patients will undergo surgical intervention for bone and joint repair and replacement. Therefore, recognizing and addressing disruptive behavior in this specialty is critical. As in other health-care settings, the barriers to eliminating this behavior from the orthopedic surgery workplace include fear of retaliation, lack of awareness among peers, and financial factors, with the associated disincentives for the system to do so.

In conclusion, it is incumbent on every health-care provider to address negative peer behavior, to contribute to improvement strategies, and to work with management to achieve team-based solutions.

TABLE 7.10. Explanations for high-risk disruptive behavior among orthopedic surgeons [7].

1. Increased patient volume
2. Decreased reimbursement
3. Increased malpractice litigation
4. Increased workplace stress
5. Job dissatisfaction

References

1. Rosenstein AH, O'Daniel M. Managing disruptive physician behavior: impact on staff relationships and patient care. Neurology. 2008;70(17):1564–70.
2. Cochran A, Elder WB. Effects of disruptive surgeon behavior in the operating room. Am J Surg. 2015;209(1):65–70.
3. Cochran A, Elder WB. A model of disruptive surgeon behavior in the perioperative environment. J Am Coll Surg. 2014;219(3): 390–8.
4. Sax HC. Building high-performance teams in the operating room. Surg Clin North Am. 2012;92(1):1519.
5. Rosenstein AH. Managing disruptive behaviors in the health care setting: focus on obstetrics services. Am J Obstet Gynecol. 2011;204(3):187–92.
6. Lyndon A, Sexton JB, Simpson KR, Rosenstein A, Lee KA, Wachter RM. Predictors of likelihood of speaking up about safety concerns in labour and delivery. BMJ Qual Saf. 2012;21(9): 791–9.
7. Patel P, Robinson BS, Novicoff VM, Dunnington GL, Brenner MJ, Saleh KJ. The disruptive orthopedic surgeon: implications for patient safety and malpractice liability. J Bone Joint Surg Am. 2011;93(21):e1261–6.

Chapter 8
Physicians in Training

Studies of disruptive behavior have recently begun to focus on troublesome conduct among resident physicians. As a basis for this evaluation, issues of professional accountability were defined by an expert consensus panel in a think tank environment [1]. The panel made the following recommendations: (1) Clear expectations should be set regarding the behavior of both faculty and residents. (2) For any behavioral deficiency cited for tracking, the desired behavior should be defined explicitly, a timeline for improvement should be set, and the consequences of continued noncompliance should be outlined clearly. (3) Health-care system problems that enable, reinforce, or perpetuate these behaviors, as an unintended consequence, should be addressed and corrected as soon as they are encountered. These are dealt with most effectively when they occur rather than at some later meeting. (4) The investigatory process should be transparent, reasonable in time and scope, and equitable to all parties involved. (5) If an intervention is warranted to address the disruptive behavior, it should be early, decisive, and monitorable (Table 8.1).

© Springer International Publishing Switzerland 2016
R.B. Vukmir, *Disruptive Healthcare Provider Behavior*,
DOI 10.1007/978-3-319-27924-4_8

TABLE 8.1. Professional accountability program for residents [1].

1. Set clear behavioral expectations
2. Define desired behavior, timeline, and consequences
3. Address systemic problems that enable behavior
4. Address issues promptly and equitably
5. Intervene early, if intervention is warranted

The panel concluded that "pursuing professional accountability" in others is most successful as an approach when one's own house is put in order first. This includes the administrative "C-suite" as well, where potentially disruptive behaviors have been known to occur in both the professional and personal arenas.

It is recognized that effective physician-to-patient communication is the cornerstone of an effective medical care program. Ravitz et al. [2] used a scripted patient communication educational module to teach family medicine trainees how to properly interview psychiatric patients. The trainees then went through a comprehensive interview review, analysis, and coaching session. Communication and self-efficacy among the study participants improved significantly in both the near and long term, after they successfully completed the instructional module and implemented it in their medical practice.

It is recognized that a physician's career development is never more heavily influenced than during his or her first year of practice. It is said that perhaps the most significant predictor of one's ultimate career trajectory is the internship year itself, which involves technical skill, teamwork, and communication.

Mullan et al. [3] performed a questionnaire-based survey of 76.4 % of 516 eligible interns concerning their exposure to disruptive behavior in their training program. They found significant agreement between attending physicians and interns (87.5 % vs. 80.4 %) that all team members performed professionally in the workplace. However, when polled, more attendings than interns felt respected in the workplace (90.0 % vs. 71.5 %, $P = 0.01$). Most of the interns (93 %) said they had experienced at least one episode of disruptive behavior, with half of them (54 %) experiencing these events at least once per month.

The adverse behaviors cited most commonly were exclusion from the decision-making process (OR, 6.97; $P < 0.001$), condescension (OR, 5.46; $P < 0.001$), and berating (OR, 4.84; $P = 0.02$). There also were reports of inappropriate jokes, abusive language, and gender bias, but these occurred at equivalent rates among both interns and attending physicians. Interestingly, although the attendings cited other physicians as the most common source of disruptive behavior, interns more commonly identified nurses (OR, 10.40; $P < 0.001$) as exhibiting this behavior.

The researchers concluded that interns experience disruptive behavior more commonly than attendings and that nurses figure prominently as a nidus of this behavior. A review of this work reveals that the most commonly cited event—omission from the decision-making process—although important in medical education, is not considered a disruptive behavior by most experts in the field.

In summary, it is crucial to realize that medical education involves a learning behavior pattern in which standards for interaction are set from the top down. The tone is set not by the institution in which one works but by the people who labor within the facility; people are more important than the "bricks and mortar."

References

1. Sanfey H, Darosa DA, Hickson GB, Williams B, Sudan R, Boehler ML, Klingensmith ME, Klamen D, Mellinger JD, Hebert JC, Richard KM, Roberts NK, Schwind CJ, Wiilliams RG, Sachdeva AK, Dinnington GL. Pursuing professional accountability: an evidence-based approach to addressing residents with behavioral problems. Arch Surg. 2012;147(7):642–7.
2. Ravitz P, Lancee WJ, Lawson A, Maunder R, Hunter JJ, Leszcz M, McNaughton N, Pain C. Improving physician-patient communication through coaching of simulated encounters. Acad Psychiatry. 2013;37(2):87–93.
3. Mullan CP, Shapiro J, McMahon GT. Intern's experiences of disruptive behavior in an academic medical center. J Grad Med Educ. 2013;5(1):25–30.

Chapter 9
Etiology

Often in cases of disruptive behavior, the provider is scrutinized first rather than the systemic issues or systematic errors and processes that may be pervasive in the health-care delivery system. More often than not, however, significant system or management issues exist as well, contributing to the aberrant behavior cited in the provider. In some cases, the examination of disruptive behavior may even go as far as a formal forensic psychiatric evaluation of the provider [1]. The typical assessment factors, both past and current performance, then are used to predict the future course. Ultimately, this approach attempts to determine the provider's fitness for duty for future endeavors. Forensic psychiatric examination often reveals psychosocial stressors and personality disorders that may be associated with these disruptive behaviors.

Roback et al. [2] attempted to delineate the personality characteristics of disruptive providers to determine whether certain personality types are predisposed to misconduct. In this study, 88 physicians were referred to the Vanderbilt Comprehensive Assessment Program for Professionals (V-CAP) for evaluation. As part of the screening process, they completed the Minnesota Multiphasic Personality Inventory-2 and/or the Personality Assessment Inventory. The participants and their subsequent behaviors were then divided into three categories: sexual boundary violations, behaviorally disruptive events, and other misconduct types. Although all three of these behaviors were viewed as potentially undesirable, the sexual boundary violators were found

© Springer International Publishing Switzerland 2016   49
R.B. Vukmir, *Disruptive Healthcare Provider Behavior*,
DOI 10.1007/978-3-319-27924-4_9

to be the greatest therapeutic challenge, with the highest treatment failure and recidivism rate.

Dang et al. [3] used the Johns Hopkins Disruptive Clinician Behavior Survey (JH-DCBS) to define and quantify disruptive clinician behavior. They performed a two-step evaluation measuring five discrete variables using focus-group analysis and a literature-based derivation set and then conducted a psychometric evaluation on a validation set of 1198 academic physicians. The authors found the profile tool to be very reliable (Cronbach's alpha, 0.79–0.91) and to have high content validity (content validity index, 0.97). They concluded that this tool provides an accurate empirical index to define and assess disruptive behavior in the workplace. The ability to define misconduct helps in developing strategies to improve the overall health-care practice environment.

Psychological dynamics are often complex in the health-care workplace, where adaptive behaviors seemingly have gone offtrack. Normally helpful behaviors that typically are associated with success may then be applied in the wrong context or situation, generating an adverse outcome. Characteristics considered productive and positive, such as intelligence and confidence, may develop into counterproductive problem traits depending on the circumstances under which they are implemented (Table 9.1) [4].

TABLE 9.1. Personality traits suggested to be found in the disruptive physician [4].

Positive traits	Negative traits	
Skilled	Arrogant	Distressing
Well read	Intimidating	Lack of insight
Rigid	Controlling	Remorseless
Dogmatic	Rigid, dogmatic	Sham apology
Hardworking	Egocentric	Lack of self-correction
Productive	Sense of entitlement	Vindictive
Confident	Lack of empathy	Litigious
Persevering	Rationalization	
Overachiever	Externalize blame	

Some theories suggest an association between disruptive provider behavior and a specific psychiatric diagnosis as described in the *Diagnostic and Statistical Manual of Mental Disorders*, fourth edition (DSM-IV) [4, 5]. The differential diagnoses associated with disruptive behavior include the more definitive Axis I principal diagnosis—specifying disease states, such as bipolar, attention deficit, intermittent explosive, and circadian rhythm disorders, as well as depression and substance use disorder. They also include more functional Axis II conditions—the personality disorders—such as borderline, narcissistic, paranoid, and passive–aggressive behavior conditions (Table 9.2). Axis III medical conditions, which imply significant chronic illness due to diabetes, as well as Axis IV social stressors, also have been implicated in disruptive behavior events.

The most recent update by the American Psychiatric Association, DSM-V, combines Axis I, II, and III conditions, suggesting that they no longer be classified as lifelong pervasive disorders [6]. The DSM update emphasizes that psychiatric illness, like any other medical disease state, can be treated effectively and cured in some cases. Therefore, the concept of associating disruptive behavior to a psychiatric diagnosis may not be a valid premise as a lifelong label.

TABLE 9.2. Psychiatric conditions associated with disruptive behavior [4, 5].

Axis I: symptom disorders
1. Attention deficit disorder
2. Bipolar disorder
3. Circadian rhythm disorder
4. Depression
5. Dementia
6. Intermittent explosive disorder
7. Substance use
Axis II: personality disorders
1. Borderline
2. Paranoid
3. Passive–aggressive
4. Narcissistic

The prototypical psychiatric diagnosis often ascribed to disruptive behavior is borderline personality disorder. In this disease state, seemingly normal societal behaviors are accentuated or are applied in the wrong context to be effective. This behavioral complex can be indicated by a triad including sexual boundary violations, alcohol issues, and substance abuse. The subtler version of this condition may manifest as attention-grabbing behaviors that are counterproductive and viewed as problematic in the health-care workplace. On the other hand, these behaviors may be viewed as well intended and directed at definitive health-care delivery issues by some.

Although reports of this type of misconduct often target staff physicians, both nursing and administrative personnel have figured prominently in these inquiries. The nursing effect is often described by other nurses, students, trainees, residents, fellows, and newer attending physicians as a manifestation of the hierarchical decision-making struggle. Moreover, disruptive behaviors by hospital administrative personnel often are accepted within a cultural code of silence based on higher rank or institutional privilege.

More commonly, misconduct among health-care personnel at any level arises from typical, organic psychological conditions, such as overwork, shift stress, burnout, and depression [7]. Therefore, this condition is dealt with more effectively by understanding the insidious progression of overwork, stress, and lack of control or input, resulting in burnout and adverse behaviors. Obviously, the goal is to improve awareness, monitoring, and prevention by offering alternative coping strategies.

References

1. Meyer DJ, Price M. Forensic psychiatric assessments of behaviorally disruptive physicians. J Am Acad Psychiatry Law. 2006;34: 72–81.
2. Roback HB, Strassberg D, Ianelli RJ, Finlayson AJ, Blanco M. Neufeld. Problematic physicians: a comparison of personality profiles by offence type. Can J Psychiatry. 2007;52(5):315–22.

3. Dang D, Nyberg D, Walrath JM, Kim MT. Development and validation of the Johns Hopkins disruptive clinician behavior survey. Am J Med Qual. 2014 Jul 28. Epub ahead of print.
4. Reynolds NT. Disruptive physician behavior: use and misuse of the label. J Med Regul. 2012;98(1):8–19.
5. American Psychiatric Association. Diagnostic manual of mental disorders. 4th ed. 2000. doi:10.1176/appi.books.9780890420249.
6. American Psychiatric Association. Diagnostic and statistical manual of mental disorders. 5th ed. 2013. doi:10.1176/appi.books.9780890425596.
7. Brown SD, Goske MJ, Johnson CM. Beyond substance abuse: stress, burnout, and depression as causes of physician impairment and disruptive behavior. J Am Coll Radiol. 2009;6(7):479–85.

Chapter 10
Nursing Interface

The most common area on which behavioral analysis has focused is the interaction between physicians and nurses. Rosenstein [1] conducted a large survey of 1200 health-care providers—physicians, nurses, and administrators—and found that the doctor–nurse relationship strongly influences nursing staff morale. The results of the survey suggest that daily interactions may have an adverse effect on nurse recruiting, job turnover, and retention at the site. Less clear, however, is who is responsible for these effects, with fingers being pointed in both directions. Because Rosenstein's study was published in a nursing journal, however, the article assigned most of the responsibility for negative interaction to the physicians.

Using the same study design, Rosenstein and O'Daniel [2] expanded the earlier analysis to a group of 1500 providers at 50 different institutions. This time, they found that equal numbers of physicians and nurses were involved in disruptive behaviors, although both groups acknowledged the adverse impact on concentration, communication, collaboration, and information transfer in the workplace. These results suggest that these behaviors not only affect staff retention but also are associated with adverse events, medical errors, patient safety, and mortality. It must be stressed, however, that this correlation with patient outcome was not proven, although it makes empiric sense.

© Springer International Publishing Switzerland 2016
R.B. Vukmir, *Disruptive Healthcare Provider Behavior*,
DOI 10.1007/978-3-319-27924-4_10

Differences between nurses and physicians regarding their perception of the consequences of misconduct have been described by others. Lyndon et al. [3] reported that compared with nurses, physicians rated potential harm in common clinical scenarios to a lesser degree. The authors found clear discrepancies in the harm ratings assigned by each of the two groups, which also correlated with the provider's likelihood of speaking up. They suggest that this disparity may explain the differences between nurses and physicians with regard to their expectations for a quality teamwork climate.

A decade later, Walrath et al. [4] used the Disruptive Clinician Behavior Survey for Hospital Settings to investigate nurses' and physicians' experiences with disruptive behavior as well as its triggers, responses, and effects on staff, patients, and the hospital. The authors found that the nurses experienced a significantly higher frequency of disruptive behavior and triggers than their physician counterparts. However, they observed a difference in perception of adverse effects, with a greater proportion of the physicians (45 % of 295) than the nurses (37 % of 689) reporting that misconduct by their peers affected them most negatively.

Overall, the survey respondents reported 189 cases of alleged patient harm as the result of disruptive behavior. Interestingly, rather than individual issues being the genesis of these behaviors, the authors found the most frequent triggers were system-related problems, such as high facility census, volume surge, and irregular patient flow scenarios. These findings should cause administrators and organizational thought leaders to take note.

Although several studies have examined the doctor–nurse interface, few have addressed its correlation with the quality of patient care. In one such study, Hutchinson and Jackson [5] analyzed 30 publications along four thematic lines: (1) physician–nurse relations and patient care; (2) nurse–nurse bullying, intimidation, and patient care; (3) reduced nurse performance related to exposure to hostile clinician behavior; and (4) nurses and physicians directly implicating patients in hostile clinician behaviors (Table 10.1). The authors also

TABLE 10.1. Themes to analyze effects of disruptive behavior [5].

1. Physician–nurse relations and patient care
2. Nurse–nurse bullying, intimidation, and patient care
3. Reduced nurse performance related to exposure to hostile clinician behaviors
4. Nurses and physicians directly implicating patients in hostile clinician behaviors

defined the forms of hostile clinician behavior that compromise nursing and patient care. Although research into disruptive behavior in the health-care setting historically has focused on physicians, these authors also noted the importance of nurse–nurse hostility and its effects on patient care. Clearly, disruptive provider behavior may involve all those participating in the health-care delivery process.

References

1. Rosenstein AH. Original research: nurse–physician relationships: impact on nurse satisfaction and retention. Am J Nurs. 2002;102(6):26–34.
2. Rosenstein AH, O'Daniel M. Disruptive behavior and clinical outcomes: perceptions of nurses and physicians. Am J Nurs. 2005;105(1):54–64.
3. Lyndon A, Sexton JB, Simpson KR, Rosenstein A, Lee KA, Wachter RM. Predictors of likelihood of speaking up about safety concerns in labour and delivery. BMJ Qual Saf. 2012;21(9):791–9.
4. Walrath JM, Dang D, Nyberg D. An organizational assessment of disruptive clinician behavior: findings and implications. J Nurs Care Qual. 2013;28(2):110–21.
5. Hutchinson M, Jackson D. Hostile clinician behaviours in the nursing work environment and implications for patient care: a mixed-methods systematic review. BMC Nurs. 2013;12(1):25.

Chapter 11
Patient Safety

Although many studies have been published describing disruptive provider behavior, finding a link to adverse effects on patient outcome has proven more elusive. Rosenstein and O'Daniel [1] reported that 67 % of the physicians and nurses they surveyed felt certain that these disruptive behaviors were linked to adverse events. Among these respondents, 71 % reported that provider misconduct led to medical errors, whereas 27 % felt it was linked to patient mortality. As with most studies, however, these findings are based on the subjective impression of the respondents as the data end point rather than objective outcome data, with defined patient morbidity and mortality. Although the authors attempted to quantify the problem of disruptive behavior in this study, their conclusion that these behaviors are linked to adverse events is based on subjective reports.

According to Felbinger [2], bullying, incivility, and similar associated disruptive behaviors are associated with significant adverse institutional effects, including employee absenteeism, job search activity, and turnover, decreased institutional commitment, and increased health-care use by the providers themselves. Factors that increase the likelihood of hostile behavior occurring include changes in hierarchy, conflicting loyalties, local stressors, and changes in medical care standards. In facilities in which this type of culture exists, management must assume the responsibility for oversight, monitoring, and intervention. More importantly, the leaders of the organization must develop and

© Springer International Publishing Switzerland 2016   59
R.B. Vukmir, *Disruptive Healthcare Provider Behavior*,
DOI 10.1007/978-3-319-27924-4_11

implement a plan that is tailored to the facility's circumstances yet feasible in light of available resources. Likewise, if an evaluation of bullying, incivility, and other disruptive behaviors uncovers any collateral information that indicates that changes are required in resource allocation or system improvement in other areas, these changes must be instituted for the program to be successful.

Another area of concern is the effect of disruptive staff interactions on providers, which manifests as a stressful health-care setting. Stecker and Stecker [3] evaluated the effect of workplace stress on the physical and psychological well-being of medical staff and whether it is linked to medical errors and suboptimal patient outcomes. They asked 617 providers to complete a Provider Conflict Questionnaire as well as a 10-item stress survey. Interestingly, most of the respondents (78.2 %) reported that the nature of the day-to-day work itself was their main stressor. The authors found the stress level was estimated to be moderate, with a mean score of 25.5 (range, 10–48), with higher stress levels noted in women. They then correlated the presence of disruptive behavior with workplace stress and found them to be almost directly proportional.

In facilities with fewer disruptive incidents, employees reported lower levels of work-related stress, whereas the converse was true in those with more disruptive behaviors, where staff reported less job satisfaction and higher workplace stress levels. The authors concluded that reducing work-related stress improves job satisfaction, resulting in decreased employee turnover; thus, stress reduction provides an economic benefit because less retraining and education are required in facilities employing staff with longer tenure. Another benefit to this type of program is a resultant environment of employee harmony and stability in which medical errors are reduced and patient care is improved.

Another aspect of disruptive provider behavior that may contribute to patient harm is a "culture of silence" in which hospital staff fear retaliation if they report misconduct. According to Mustard [4], if the culture of silence is accepted, it may result in a "history of tolerance and indifference to intimidating and destructive behaviors." These behaviors may range from overt acts, such as shouting or use of profanity, to more passive acts regarding call response, documentation, or punctuality. The key to avoiding a culture of silence is to acknowledge and confront the behavior, often using multidisciplinary teams consisting of physicians, nurses, and therapists, as well as outside experts skilled in health-care wellness, to facilitate program success.

Leape [5], one of the originators of early theories on patient safety, and colleagues have suggested that times of "frustratingly slow progress" may be a result of the protected, isolated nature of established patient care processes and procedures. In their work, they describe the medical ethos and hierarchical structure of institutionalized medicine that discourages transparency and information sharing among groups. The Lucian Leape Institute, established by the US National Patient Safety Foundation, identified five pillars of a successful patient safety program: transparency, care integration, patient/consumer integration, restoration of joy and meaning at work, and medical education reform (Table 11.1) [5]. The institute believes a system incorporating these concepts will result in meaningful improvements in health care.

As pointed out earlier, however, attempts to quantify provider misconduct in the health-care workplace have not been a complete success. Saxton et al. [6] investigated the impact of nurse–physician disruptive behavior on patient safety by reviewing ten articles identified by the keyword *disruptive physician behavior* and reported that all the studies were

TABLE 11.1. Five requirements of a successful patient safety program [5].

1. System transparency
2. Health-care integration
3. Patient/consumer engagement
4. Restoration of joy and meaning at work
5. Medical education reform

descriptive in nature and used nonexperimental approaches and self-report methodology rather than quantitative outcome end points. Although the authors found that disruptive behavior is alarmingly prevalent, they acknowledged the limitations of the study approach and concluded that a standard definition for disruptive behavior is needed for the topic to be examined effectively.

Despite all the efforts and attention focused on provider misbehavior and its impact on patient safety, the success of programs instituted to address this problem varies widely. As noted by Rosenstein [7], it is well known that disruptive behavior adversely affects relationships, collaboration, communication, and process flow, subsequently compromising patient care. He recommends quality and safety awareness programs, policies, procedures, and educational programs to hold individuals accountable as well as remediation programs to correct disruptive behavior. It is crucial to remember that when professional misconduct is encountered, attention must be focused not only on the individual but also on the systemic and resource deficiencies that may have triggered it. Still lacking in the scientific community is a research model to directly tie disruptive behaviors to patient outcomes.

References

1. Rosenstein AH, O'Daniel M. A survey of the impact of disruptive behaviors and communication defects on patient safety. Jt Comm J Qual Patient Saf. 2008;34(8):464–71.
2. Felbinger DM. Bullying, incivility and disruptive behaviors in the healthcare setting: identification, impact and intervention. Front Health Serv Manage. 2009;25(4):13–23.
3. Stecker M, Stecker MM. Disruptive staff interactions: a serious source of inter-provider conflict and stress in health care settings. Issues Ment Health Nurs. 2014;35(7):533–41.
4. Mustard LW. The culture of silence: disruptive and impaired physicians. J Med Pract Manage. 2009;25(3):153–5.

5. Leape L, Berwick D, Clancy C, Gluck P, Guest J, Lawrence D, Morath J, O'Leary D, O'Neill P, Pinakiewicz D, Isaac T. Transforming healthcare: a safety imperative. Qual Saf Health Care. 2009;18:424–8.
6. Saxton R, Hines T, Enriquez M. The negative impact of nurse-physician disruptive behavior on patient safety: a review of the literature. J Patient Saf. 2009;5(3):180–3.
7. Rosenstein AH. The quality and economic impact of disruptive behaviors on clinical outcome of patient care. Am J Med Qual. 2011;26(5):372–9.

Chapter 12
Policy and Guidelines

The basis of any program dealing with disruptive behavior is the institution of a disruptive conduct policy or guideline, which should be widely understood and supported by all team members involved [1]. The first step in this process is to establish structures and systems to define and communicate what constitutes unacceptable behavior. Second, a clear pathway should be set up for staff members to follow if they encounter this type of behavior in the workplace. Third, the program should support an overall institutional focus on promoting a sustainable, healthy work environment (Table 12.1).

An oft-cited quandary is whether the problem rests with the individual or the system. Historically, administrative staff has had a tendency to blame the provider, whereas providers blame other departments or the system. Thought leaders in this field, such as Leape and Fromson [2], have a fairly physician-centric view regarding the etiology of disruptive behavior in the health-care arena. Their 2006 treatise postulates that first, performance failure among physicians is "not a rare phenomenon" when its incidence is described qualitatively. Second, disruptive behavior poses a substantial threat to the welfare of the facility and the safety of patients. Third, few hospitals have the capability to respond to these incidents promptly and effectively with the expertise required to truly achieve success. Often, a local "expert" is appointed as a de facto leader, although he or she may have little formal training in the analysis, intervention, and remediation process.

© Springer International Publishing Switzerland 2016   65
R.B. Vukmir, *Disruptive Healthcare Provider Behavior*,
DOI 10.1007/978-3-319-27924-4_12

TABLE 12.1. Instituting a disruptive conduct policy [1].

1. Establish a structure to define the disruptive behavior
2. Ensure the policy is followed when behavior is encountered
3. Include systems to promote a healthy work environment

TABLE 12.2. Issues regarding a system-level solution to poor physician performance [2].

1. Physician performance failure is not rare
2. Disruptive behavior poses a threat to public welfare and safety
3. Individual hospitals do not have systems in place to respond
4. Failure to monitor is a breach of fiduciary duty
5. National or state standards of conduct or competence or measures to monitor performance are lacking

Fourth, the medical profession's failure to monitor physician quality and performance according to set standards is a breach of its fiduciary responsibility to the public. Fifth, a hospital's failure to deal with unprofessional conduct adequately often is the result of the absence of state and/or local standards for measuring performance and for identifying and correcting disruptive behavior in the workplace (Table 12.2).

The authors concluded that most hospitals are not capable of dealing with this issue locally and that a national effort is needed to provide them with the resources and expertise needed to assist in the process. They identified several organizations that already have a fiduciary responsibility to the general public in ensuring competent, safe care and that are best positioned to take on this task. These include the Federation of State Medical Boards, the American Board of Medical Specialties, and the Joint Commission on Accreditation of Healthcare Organizations, all of which have the capacity to assist in the monitoring and intervention process. However, the Joint Commission now requires each institution to develop its own program to deal with disruptive behavior. A criticism of this analysis is that its focus on physicians may be extreme. Furthermore, the organizations cited indeed have a responsibility but a much broader one than previously thought.

The nebulous nature of the disruptive behavior problem as well as potential solutions may require innovative techniques, and attempts have been made to develop computer modeling programs to assist in this endeavor. Piper [3] proposed a theoretic model using a scenario-based system to provide solutions to a series of internal conflict gamuts and profiles. The author concluded that a workplace culture with less internal conflict is more likely to achieve its quality patient care objectives.

The Joint Commission mandates that health-care leaders develop "a code of conduct that defines acceptable behavior and behaviors that undermine a culture of safety" [4]. This mandate also includes a requirement for tracking, analyzing, monitoring, and managing these behaviors. It is recognized that rules and standards are an effective approach to promote quality and safety; however, physicians' associations have advised their members to familiarize themselves with their facility's disruptive behavior program and to monitor its implementation process to prevent abuse. The Wisconsin Medical Society, for example, cautions its members to be wary of vague definitions, encroachments on their rights, staff privileging requirements, and most importantly, the misuse of the code of conduct memorialized in medical staff bylaws [5]. The physician must take an active role in protecting his or her own rights while advocating for his or her patients as well as for all members of the health-care team.

The key to the successful implementation of a disruptive behavior policy is mutual trust. The best way to ensure that goal is for all parties to reach as much consensus as possible in drafting the particular document. The ideal disruptive behavior policy or protocol should be as specific and well defined as possible. Typically, it begins with an introductory statement outlining the policy's goals and objectives. This is followed by a section defining the types and format of offensive behavior, then a series of examples of those behaviors. Next, the document provides a detailed protocol for reporting, documenting, and analyzing the behavior, as well as an action plan that lists the protections and safeguards in place while the issue is being resolved.

An especially important component of a good disruptive behavior protocol is a severity index to classify the incident. The document also typically includes a due process protocol elucidating the recommended steps toward resolution. Finally, the document concludes by identifying an educational or remediation component. Typically, for a plan to be successful, it must be transparent and include explicit policies or protocols with identifiable, objective parameters to facilitate provider participation.

References

1. Barnsteiner JH, Madigan C, Spray TL. Instituting a disruptive conduct policy for medical staff. AACN Clin Issues. 2001;12(3):378–82.
2. Leape LL, Fromson JA. Problem doctors: is there a system level solution. Ann Intern Med. 2006;144(2):107–15.
3. Piper LE. A theoretical model to address organizational human conflict and disruptive behavior in health care organizations. Health Care Manag. 2006;25(4):315–20.
4. Joint Commission Perspectives. Revision to LD.03.01.01, EPs 4 and 5. Jt Comm Accredit Healthc Organ. 2012;32(1):7.
5. Leiker M. Sentinel events, disruptive behavior and medical staff codes of conduct. WMJ. 2009;108(6):333–4.

Chapter 13
Economic Issues

It is widely believed that disruptive behaviors have a negative impact on staff relationships, team collaboration, communication, patient flow, and staff efficiency, resulting in worsened patient outcomes [1]. However, they also have been associated with problems in revenue cycling, cost structure, and financial performance. Rosenstein [1] suggested that because of local loyalties and sympathies, institutions are more willing to address system improvements to improve patient safety than to tackle human impact issues, such as professional misconduct. He proposed a strategic plan to address the adverse quality and economic effects of disruptive behaviors based on the following ten steps: (1) establish a defined organizational leadership strategy; (2) stress awareness and accountability at all levels of the organization; (3) recognize that general education is the key to the current and future success of the program; (4) target focused, specialized education to a particular area or issue; (5) become especially facile with the use of various communication and collaboration tools; (6) realize that the key to success is proper champion identification and facilitation; (7) ensure that comprehensive operational policies and procedures are developed and maintained; (8) define and implement the details of the incident-reporting process; (9) once an issue is defined, determine how the intervention is implemented successfully; and (10) garner institutional support for patient safety, quality, and risk management programs, which is the most crucial step.

© Springer International Publishing Switzerland 2016
R.B. Vukmir, *Disruptive Healthcare Provider Behavior*,
DOI 10.1007/978-3-319-27924-4_13

Subsequently, Rosenstein [2] published another call to action to address the economic impact of disruptive behaviors as well as their overall effect on health-care quality. He suggested that institutions indeed recognize the full spectrum of the impact of misconduct on the health-care delivery process. Too often, however, classic remediation programs target only the misbehavior, focusing on policies, education, awareness, accountability, and training to address negative behaviors. Organizations also should take positive approaches to improve team communication and collaboration to improve the quality of care.

With the advent of rising expenses and decreasing reimbursements, institutions have looked toward disruptive behavior as a potential area to achieve cost savings. Rawson et al. [3] evaluated costs at a 400-bed hospital and studied the economic impact of disruptive behavior. They estimated that staff turnover, as well as medication and procedural errors, costs the institution in excess of $1 million. The authors concluded that redirecting these resources within an academic medical center could improve patient safety, reduce medical errors, and improve student and resident education.

One way to lessen the economic impact of disruptive behavior is to minimize employee turnover, which is an area of potentially controllable cost. Clearly, in the era of declining reimbursement, financial viability often hinges on cost control. McCracken et al. [4] proposed a list of ten personality traits of the disruptive physician that might be related to future performance, as defined by an adverse behavior end point. They then described the behaviors that might be used to assist in identifying trends, providing information they believe to be useful in making hiring decisions down the road. The authors defined the projected markers of problematic behaviors and their effect on peer interaction to include these correlates (Table 13.1).

The most significant trait of disruptive physicians is their inability to get along with peers, colleagues, and coworkers, which manifests as difficulty in participating cooperatively in group practice patterns, protocols, and guidelines. Second,

TABLE 13.1. Personality traits associated with disruptive behavior [4].

1. Difficulty in getting along with peers and colleagues
2. Coworker difficulty
3. Not successful in group practice
4. Problems with protocols and guidelines
5. Decreased sociability and trust
6. Poor group goal sharing
7. Cooperative team approach struggles
8. Impulsive behavior and poor self-control
9. Aggressive behavior
10. Unyielding in goal attainment

this group has demonstrable difficulties with sociability, trust, and group goal sharing in their professional interactions. This manifests most often when a cooperative team approach and partnership are required to meet the institutional goals and objectives established for program success. Third, this group often exhibits high degrees of impulsive behavior and poor self-control when confronted by stressful situations. They often act aggressively and are unyielding with regard to goal attainment.

It is important to remember, however, that the difference between desirable and undesirable behavior often is only a matter of degree, circumstances, and timing. At times, the local administration may lose its focus on the mission (Table 13.2) and require input and oversight by the board of directors to maintain its objectivity.

Holloway and Kusy [5] examined the effect of disruptive and toxic behaviors on the health-care bottom line, describing "uncivil behaviors" that lead to absenteeism and threaten workplace productivity, worker motivation, and the physical and emotional well-being of the health-care providers involved in these events. According to the authors, the three toxic behaviors that have the greatest detrimental effect in the health-care workplace are shaming, passive hostility, and team sabotage. The quantitative effects of these behaviors

TABLE 13.2. Ten components to address disruptive behavior [1].

1. Organizational leadership
2. Awareness and accountability
3. Education
4. Special education
5. Communication and collaboration tools
6. Clinical champion
7. Policies and procedures
8. Reporting process
9. Intervention process
10. Patient safety, quality, risk programs

TABLE 13.3. Quantitative effects of toxic behavior [5, 6].

Effect	Incidence (%)
Time lost worrying	80
Organizational commitment decline	78
Performance decline	68
Avoidance time	63
Decreased work effort	48
Decreased work time	47
Decreased work quality	38
Job resignation	12

were defined by Pearson and Porath [6] and summarized by Holloway [5], who reported the following demonstrable impact of toxic behavior on other personnel: 12 % of victims quit outright, 48 % decreased their work effort, 47 % decreased productive work time, 38 % decreased work quality, 68 % reported subjective work performance decline, 80 % lost time worrying about the issue, 63 % spent time avoiding the problem, and 78 % felt their commitment to the organization declined (Table 13.3).

The key here is to recognize that any staff member may leave a toxic environment. In a geographic area that offers many job opportunities, many providers often do exactly that, whereas workers with more limited opportunities will accept more workplace dysfunction. The expense of repeated hiring, rehiring, training, and orienting can be minimized in a stable, healthy work environment.

References

1. Rosenstein AH. Measuring and managing the economic impact of disruptive behaviors in the hospital. J Healthc Risk Manag. 2010;30(2):20–6.
2. Rosenstein AH. The quality and economic impact of disruptive behaviors on clinical outcome of patient care. Am J Med Qual. 2011;26(5):372–9.
3. Rawson JV, Thompson N, Sostre G, Deitte L. The cost of disruptive and unprofessional behaviors in health care. Acad Radiol. 2013;20(9):2074–6.
4. McCracken J, Hicks R. Personality traits of a disruptive physician. Physician Exec. 2012;38(5):66–8.
5. Holloway EL, Kusy M. Disruptive and toxic behaviors in healthcare: zero tolerance, the bottom line, and what to do about it. J Med Pract Manage. 2010;25(6):335–40.
6. Pearson CM, Porath CL. On the nature, consequences and remedies of workplace incivility: no time for "nice"? Think again. Acad Manage Exec. 2005;19(1):7–18.

Chapter 14
Legal Interface

One of the first authors to address the legal implications of disruptive behavior was Purtell [1] more than three decades ago. He described a scenario in which facilities were just beginning to tackle this sensitive issue. At that time, 22 % of states (11) had statutory guidelines allowing hospitals to dismiss physicians demonstrating disruptive behavior. Even back then, facilities were warned to be careful when documenting a correlation between professional misconduct and an adverse effect on patient care to avoid subsequent litigation. Because of the ease with which bias sometimes enters an analysis, they were encouraged to seek objective, quantifiable evidence of harm.

As with most legal conflicts, the adversarial process is especially disadvantageous in reviewing medical staff disputes [2]. These events are time consuming and costly and disrupt medical staff–hospital relationships, which may impose an added burden in trying times. Patients often suffer as well when an issue is resolved in an adversarial setting. Therefore, an alternative dispute resolution (ADR) approach was suggested as an alternative to litigation. ADR uses shared decision-making to find mutually agreeable solutions, minimizing the harm to established parties and relationships.

The legal standard for this analysis returns to the benchmarks established by national regulatory organizations, such as the

© Springer International Publishing Switzerland 2016
R.B. Vukmir, *Disruptive Healthcare Provider Behavior*,
DOI 10.1007/978-3-319-27924-4_14

Joint Commission, and other professional societies, such as the American Medical Association (AMA), that routinely provide oversight and advice on matters such as these [3–6].

Joint Commission Leadership Standard LD.3.10, established in 2009, defines the obligations of the health-care system to confront disruptive behavior through elements of performance (EP) and medical staff (MS) provisions [3, 4]. These obligations include EP.4, which requires facilities to establish a code of conduct defining proper, unacceptable, and prohibited behaviors. This obligation is extended by EP.5, which requires leaders to institute a process to evaluate and manage disruptive behavior at their institution.

The medical staff oversight section (MS.4) mandates that six core competencies be factored into the initial and ongoing medical staff credentialing process: (1) patient care, (2) medical/clinical knowledge, (3) practice-based learning and improvement, (4) interpersonal and communication skills, (5) professionalism, and (6) system-based practice (Table 14.1). These requirements are now a routine part of the medical staff credentialing process for all health-care institutions and are incorporated in both the Ongoing Professional Practice Evaluation (OPPE) and the Focused Professional Practice Evaluation (FPPE). The OPPE is performed regularly and routinely as a screening tool to evaluate providers on medical staff as part of the ongoing credentialing process, whereas the FPPE is used on an as-needed basis to follow-up with providers identified by the OPPE as potentially delivering a substandard level of care.

TABLE 14.1. The Joint Commission's core competencies for physicians [4].

1. Patient care
2. Medical/clinical knowledge
3. Practice-based learning and improvement
4. Interpersonal and communication skills
5. Professionalism
6. System-based practice

The six core competencies also have been incorporated by individual medical specialty boards into their ongoing Maintenance of Certification (MOC) programs.

To define an institution's obligations regarding disruptive physician behavior in the health-care workplace, the AMA established Policy H-140.918 [5, 6]. This guideline defines disruptive behavior as any professional conduct, either physical or verbal, that may affect patient care in a negative way. It recommends that each medical staff develop and adopt bylaws for the identification, intervention, and referral of this behavior to an appropriate wellness committee. This policy should strive for maximal specificity by setting explicit criteria to define behaviors and subsequent actions.

The most commonly invoked "legal" intervention is a forensic psychiatric assessment of the physician alleged to have engaged in disruptive behavior (Table 14.2) [7]. The first-level remedy for this type of behavior is for the provider to attend a continuing medical education (CME) "boundary" course. The crossing of certain boundaries by professionals may or may not be acceptable outside the hospital setting but clearly is appropriate in the health-care facility. Therefore, these CME courses, which typically provide 12–25 h of credit, instruct the provider on the proper delineation of professional boundaries that must honored in the health-care setting. This approach commonly is used for referrals who have exhibited milder forms of disruptive behavior.

More severe allegations of behavioral disruption are addressed by referring the provider to a psychiatrist or other clinician for forensic examination. This assessment usually is intensive and performed by a multidisciplinary team.

TABLE 14.2. Forensic psychiatric assessment [7].

1. Physician boundary course
2. Forensic psychiatric assessment
3. Diagnosis—behavioral, psychiatric, medical
4. Current "fitness for duty"
5. Future recidivism potential

The goals of forensic examination differ from those of the typical civil adjudication process in that proximate cause and patient harm are not essential elements raised by the examiner. Rather, the examiner evaluates the facts of the case by interviewing the examinee, as well as witnesses, and reports the findings to the agency requesting the examination, typically a medical board or facility. The examiner often makes a diagnosis, including behavioral, psychiatric, and medical aspects, and gives his or her opinion on whether the provider is fit for present and future duties as well as what treatment or monitoring may be needed to ensure the provider fulfills those professional capacities. This task is difficult, but not impossible, as there is experience with both success and recidivism rates.

The court system also has allowed us to process definitions of disruptive behavior into workable models to aid our understanding. Court rulings have established applicable standards and thresholds for nonrenewal, modification, or revocation of staff privileges [8]. However, it is important for the physician to recognize that judicial authorities have given health-care facilities a fairly wide berth in defining and acting on professional misconduct. Moreover, the *disruptive* label sometimes has been applied to providers attempting to illustrate and improve aberrant medical care, staffing, or operational issues. However, a physician's peers often are best at defining intent and are essential in helping resolve the problem. Little due process is afforded to medical staff physicians in hospital bylaws.

The *disruptive* label often is invoked even when no actual standard-of-care issues have been identified. However, the courts typically grant immunity to facilities in their self-policing of staff privileging decisions. They assume the hospital has the knowledge and capability to make the proper decisions, so they distance themselves from the details and factual analysis. Therefore, only the most egregious cases of alleged financial misdoing, competitive disadvantage, or discriminatory intent rise to the level of judicial resolution in the favor of the physician.

References

1. Purtell DJ. How to deal with the disruptive physician. Hosp Med Staff. 1981;10(1):10–4.
2. Hall Jr JL, Strong RA. Alternative dispute resolution and the physician—the use of mediation to resolve hospital-medical staff conflicts. Med Staff Couns. 1993;7(2):1–7.
3. AMA. AMA Code of Medical Ethics. Opinion 9.045—physicians with disruptive behavior. 2000. http://www.ama-assn.org/ama/pub/physician-resources/medical-ethics/code-medical-ethics/opinion9045.page. Accessed 4 Mar 2012.
4. The Joint Commission. Sentinel event alert: behaviors that undermine a culture of safety. 2008;(Issue 40). www.jointcommission.org/SentinelEvents/SentinelEventAlert/sea_40.htm. Accessed 20 Sept 2010.
5. Joint Commission Perspectives. Revision to LD.03.01.01, EPs 4 and 5. Jt Comm Accredit Healthc Organ. 2012;32(1):7.
6. Anderson G, Anderson B. JCAHO changes the term "disruptive behavior" as it relates to physicians. Anderson and Anderson. Nov 29, 2011.
7. Meyer DM, Price M. Forensic psychiatric assessments of behaviorally disruptive physicians. J Am Acad Psychiatry Law. 2006;34:72–81.
8. Grogan MJ, Knechtges P. The disruptive physician: a legal perspective. Acad Radiol. 2013;20(9):1069–73. https://www.andersonservices.com/blog/2011/11/jcaho-changes-the-term-disruptive-behavior-as-it-relatestophysicans/

Chapter 15
Regulatory Interventions

Most of the legal interventions in cases of professional misconduct are fraught with difficulty for all parties involved; therefore, other alternatives have emerged that bring together various regulatory agencies and programs. The provision of medical malpractice insurance ostensibly is another marker of quality as well as a means to control physician behavior.

Schwartz and Mendelson [1] examined 920 providers who had lost their medical malpractice coverage as some consequence of their practice. They found that some specialties were overrepresented in this group, especially obstetrics/gynecology (21 %) and family practice (16 %). There was also an overrepresentation regarding age, with the largest cohort made up of those aged 45–54 years. The authors found no correlation between loss of insurance and specialty board certification; likewise, physicians who received their medical training in the United States and those who were educated in other countries were equally represented in the study group (Table 15.1).

© Springer International Publishing Switzerland 2016
R.B. Vukmir, *Disruptive Healthcare Provider Behavior*,
DOI 10.1007/978-3-319-27924-4_15

TABLE 15.1. Loss of medical malpractice insurance overview [1].

1. Specialties at risk: obstetrics/gynecology (21 %), family medicine (16 %)
2. Age cohort: 45–54 years
3. Board certification: no correlation
4. Medical school, domestic or international: no correlation

TABLE 15.2. State medical board disciplinary actions [2].

Behavior	Incidence (%)
Negligence or incompetence	34
Alcohol or drug abuse	14
Inappropriate prescribing practice	11
Inappropriate contact	10
Fraud	9
Overall incidence	0.24

Clearly, from the underwriter's perspective, disruptive behavior may result in a provider being refused coverage based on the loss of medical staff privileges or medical licensure.

Morrison and Wickersham [2] reported on another risk cohort: physicians who have been disciplined by a state medical board. In their evaluation of 375 practicing physicians, they discovered that 0.24 % were the subject of disciplinary actions. The most frequent reasons for action were negligence or incompetence (34 %), alcohol or drug abuse (14 %), inappropriate prescribing practice (11 %), inappropriate contact (10 %), and outright fraud (9 %) (Table 15.2). The authors also found a demographic component to disciplinary actions imposed by medical licensing boards, with a higher incidence among providers with a greater number of direct patient encounters (OR, 2.56) and those with more years of practice, typically more than 20 (OR, 2.02). However, they found a lower incidence among female physicians (OR, 0.44) and board-certified providers (OR, 0.42) (Table 15.3).

TABLE 15.3. Disciplinary action demographic profile [3].

Factor	Incidence (OR)
Higher	
1. Patient care encounters	2.56
2. Length of practice (>20 years)	2.02
Lower	
3. Female gender	0.44
4. Board certification	0.42

Typically, the responsibility for physician censuring rests with the state medical boards, which may recommend no action, education, practice limitation, or probation or may revoke the doctor's license outright.

Another important regulatory intervention is analysis by a hospital peer-review committee, which then reports its findings to the National Practitioner Data Bank (NPDB). Baldwin et al. [3] conducted a retrospective cohort study of reports to the NPDB between 1991 and 1995 from 4743 hospitals and found an overall reporting rate of 2.26 (range 0.40–52.3) per 100,000 admissions. A subgroup analysis revealed that the proportion of hospitals reporting an action decreased from 11.6 % in 1991 to 10.0 % in 1995. It also found a higher incidence of reporting by urban hospitals versus rural ones (OR, 1.21) and a lower incidence in teaching hospitals (OR, 0.54).

Finally, although they typically are focused on quality of care, quality committees also appear to be well suited to handling reports of professional misconduct.

References

1. Schwartz WB, Mendelson DN. Physicians who have lost their malpractice insurance. JAMA. 1989;262(10):1335–41.
2. Morrison J, Wickersham P. Physician disciplined by a State Medical Board. JAMA. 1998;279(23):1889–93.
3. Baldwin LM, Hart LG, Oshel RE, Fordyce MA, Cohen R, Rosenblatt RA. Hospital peer review and the National Practitioner Data Bank: clinical privileges action reports. JAMA. 1999;282(4):349–55.

Chapter 16
Strategies for Improvement

An essential skill for efficient and effective operations is the ability to resolve conflict.

As Kennedy [1] proposes in her article "A Crash Course in Conflict Resolution," there are four main sources of conflict that occur in the workplace (Table 16.1): (1) real or imagined differences in values; (2) dissimilar goals and objectives, which often may inhibit teamwork and cooperation; (3) poor communication between parties, which often exacerbates minor differences, resulting in unsolvable dilemmas; and (4) overpersonalization of generic or organizational issues. The goal is to encourage participation and buy-in by all parties; however, too much attachment to a project sometimes may be counterproductive as well. Ideally, goal sharing benefits the patients, whereas any benefits to the providers should be shared equally.

The cornerstone of success in conflict resolution is to arrive at a mutually agreeable solution, not a one-sided approach to the problem (Table 16.2) [1]. This process requires three steps: (1) differences in values among the stakeholders must be addressed at the beginning of the project, (2) effective communication styles must be established to ensure that all parties contribute equally to the dialogue, and (3) everyone must commit to a mutually satisfactory resolution of the issues in play. Once these tasks are accomplished, the group's ability to move forward is much more likely to occur.

Insidious costs accrue as a result of the pervasive stress associated with disruptive physician behavior [2]. Misconduct

© Springer International Publishing Switzerland 2016
R.B. Vukmir, *Disruptive Healthcare Provider Behavior*,
DOI 10.1007/978-3-319-27924-4_16

TABLE 16.1. Sources of workplace conflict [1].

1. Real or perceived differences in values
2. Dissimilar goals and objectives
3. Poor communication
4. Personalization of generic or organizational issues

TABLE 16.2. Steps toward conflict resolution [1].

1. Address value differences
2. Establish effective communication techniques
3. Make sure everyone is committed to success

TABLE 16.3. Costs of pervasive workplace stress [2].

1. Acceleration of organizational turnover
2. Shift in focus away from productive activity
3. Greater likelihood of substandard practice
4. Stress among colleagues

in the workplace can undermine the morale of the practice, accelerating employee turnover, diverting focus from productive activities, increasing the likelihood of substandard care, and creating tension among colleagues (Table 16.3). An effective manager knows how to confront and manage disruptive behavior to achieve workplace harmony while ensuring the practitioner exhibiting this conduct is rehabilitated.

To address the problem of disruptive provider behavior, organizational leaders need to develop a system to prevent or reduce this behavior and to rehabilitate providers labeled as "disruptive" (Table 16.4) [2]. Suggested strategies include the following: (1) what constitutes reasonable and competent interpersonal behavior should be clearly defined. Staff should then be encouraged to go above and beyond that benchmark every day. (2) Staff should be educated on the interpersonal skill set required for an effective medical practice. (3) A method for evaluating and comparing interpersonal skills should be implemented. (4) A policy should be established

TABLE 16.4. Steps in developing a system to address behavior [2].

1. Define reasonable and competent interpersonal behavior
2. Provide education on interpersonal skills
3. Develop a method to evaluate interpersonal skills
4. Develop a policy and procedures
5. Assess and confront the behavior
6. Rehabilitate the individual

TABLE 16.5. Seven steps to resolve the disruptive physician behavior problem [3].

1. Provide protection to "complainants"
2. Listen, empathize, and avoid communication triangles
3. Confront "offenders" with authority, compassion, and data
4. Obtain outside assistance from experts when necessary
5. Offer workplace training and education to foster positive experiences
6. Follow up on all interventions
7. Practice what you preach

that clearly describes the process for managing disruptive behavior. (5) Most importantly, a process should be developed to assess and confront the behavior and to rehabilitate the individual whose behavior is deemed disruptive. Perhaps instead of emphasizing negative behaviors, it would be more effective to define and emulate the positive behaviors required for success.

Managing workplace conflict is one of the most significant, stressful, and time-consuming aspects of a hospital administrator's responsibility [3]. The key is to understand the organization's interpersonal dynamics and to foster a positive environment to effect tangible, lasting institutional change. Lastly, one must truly "walk the walk" to have credibility among one's peers, colleagues, and coworkers.

In an attempt to solve the disruptive physician dilemma, Sotile and Sotile [3] proposed a seven-step approach (Table 16.5). Step 1 is to establish unequivocal protections for the "complainants," so staff members are not hesitant in reporting misconduct out of fear of retaliation. Step 2 is to hear the entire story before commenting, to empathize, and to avoid communication triangles. Direct, first-person communication is always best to ensure accuracy; relying on hearsay and reports of others may be problematic. Step 3 is to "confront the offender" authoritatively but compassionately. Clearly, citing data specific to the individual case, under the customary protections, is more effective than citing generalities concerning the event. Step 4 is to seek outside help from experts, if necessary, for complex matters or when a higher degree of objectivity or authoritative control is required. Step 5 is to offer workplace training, continuing education, and instruction that engender positive experiences for all involved personnel. Step 6 is to ensure adequate follow-up of all interventions aimed at correcting the disruptive behavior. Finally, step 7 is for physician leaders to "practice what they preach," which is recognized as a common theme among several authorities.

This process of self-assessment, comprehensive thinking, and advanced planning will help health-care executives move their organizations forward. Thus, they will be able to transition from a reactionary mode of conflict management to a system that can withstand the extraordinary challenges of today's health-care system on a day-to-day basis.

The cornerstones of a successful medical practice are good working relationships and a happy workplace environment; yet, in a significant number of cases, the opposite scenario exists. Strained work relationships may be associated stress, resulting in errors and patient harm and potentially affecting the facility's bottom line. Hills [4] developed a staff training tool consisting of 50 specific strategies allowing employees to build relationships with the physicians with whom they work. These recommendations emphasize a team approach, stressing the importance of harmonious interaction within a multidisciplinary health-care provider team.

Vanderbilt University School of Medicine (VUSM) has a comprehensive program in place to teach professionalism to its faculty and staff. In addition, Hickson et al. [5] described VUSM's complementary approach to identify, measure, and address unprofessional behavior. The key elements of this program are a commitment by leaders to address professional misconduct, a model to guide intervention, supportive institutional policies, surveillance tools to capture patient and staff complaints, a review process, multilevel training, and resources to address disruptive behavior (Table 16.6).

VUSM's model for dealing with disruptive behavior focuses on four graduated, progressive interventions to assist in the rehabilitative program [5]. The first step addresses "single unprofessional incidents" and includes an informal conversation with the provider, even if he or she is the subject of only one report of misbehavior. If data reveal a pattern of disruptive behavior, the second step is an "awareness intervention" in which this information is shared with the provider in a nonpunitive manner. If the disruptive pattern persists, the third step—the authority intervention—comes into play. This intervention requires the facility's leaders to develop and implement an improvement and evaluation plan for the physician. If the provider fails to respond to the authority intervention, the fourth step is formal disciplinary action (Table 16.7).

The VUSM program has been successful for several reasons. First, all physicians are involved in peer counseling, whereas physician leaders receive additional training for higher-level intervention. The best way to learn how to improve one's own behavior is to evaluate others. Second, instead of following a single strategy, the program takes a "balance beam" approach, weighing the advantages and

TABLE 16.6. Elements of the VUSM professionalism program [5].

1. Leadership commitment
2. Model to guide intervention
3. Supportive institutional policies
4. Surveillance tools
5. Review processes
6. Multilevel training
7. Resources to address behavior

TABLE 16.7. Graduated disruptive behavior action plan [5].

1. Informal conversation for single incidents
2. Nonpunitive awareness interventions when patterns emerge
3. Leader-developed action plans when patterns persist
4. Imposition of disciplinary process if previous steps fail

TABLE 16.8. Vanderbilt professionalism program's keys to success [5].

1. Involves all physicians in informal peer counseling
2. Provides physician leaders with additional training for higher-level intervention
3. Uses a balance beam rather than a single-solution approach
4. Acknowledges barriers to success: excuses, denial, rationalization
5. Performs constant surveillance to decrease incidence

disadvantages of alternative strategies. Third, understanding and redirecting common excuses, rationalizations, denials, and barriers to change make physicians more effective in their therapeutic role. Fourth, the program's consistent interventional approach prevents the resurgence of adverse behavioral patterns. Fifth, the emphasis on a professional workplace environment leads to improvements in job satisfaction, patient safety, and the institution's reputation, both externally and internally (Table 16.8).

To address disruptive behavior and incivility in the health-care workplace, Holloway and Kusy [6] presented a model they call the Toxic Organization Change System (TOCS). This program uses a tripartite approach addressing the individual, the team, and the organization to ensure success (Table 16.9). At the individual level, the model includes a performance appraisal process that sets clear expectations regarding civility and collects consistent, systematic feedback from key stakeholders that may be used to develop an individualized set of objectives for behavioral change. In other words, the key is to use the performance appraisal process to determine individual expectations, which may be used as a screening tool for at-risk personnel (Table 16.10).

TABLE 16.9. Strategies of the TOCS model [6].

1. Individual level
A. Performance management
Value civility
B. Systematic feedback
2. Team level
A. Integration of civility values into team norm
B. 360-degree team assessment
C. Identification of toxic protectors and buffers
3. Organizational strategies
A. Policy of respectful engagement
B. Core value benchmarks
Performance management
Leadership development

TABLE 16.10. Steps in the performance appraisal process [6].

1. Assemble feedback from key stakeholders
2. Establish target-specific definition for toxic behavior
3. Establish timeline for periodic progress review
4. Have individuals develop their own professional growth goals
5. Define criteria for respectful engagement

This process uses feedback to set goals to be met on an established timeline while emphasizing professional growth and respectful engagement.

At the team level, one strategy is to apply the values of civility to the everyday work environment, thus incorporating them in the team's norms. Another strategy important for the group's functioning is "360-degree team assessment," in which the team members and supervisors evaluate each other. However, although this approach is meant to improve supervisory performance, it often is limited to midlevel managers, excluding the upper echelon of the institution. Finally, Holloway and Kusy [6] identified two team roles: toxic protectors, who, out of self-interest, protect the individual exhibiting the disruptive behavior, and toxic buffers, who protect and insulate their teammates from the disruptive individual. These team members inadvertently perpetuate uncivil conduct in the workplace and prolong the situation by hiding the behaviors from those who have the authority to take corrective action. As an intervention, the authors suggest providing feedback to toxic protectors and buffers to make them aware of how their actions are contributing to an uncivil environment.

At the organizational level, the overarching strategy is to define specific behaviors that contribute to an atmosphere of respectful engagement. These benchmarks then are integrated into performance management and leadership development activities and become part of the performance appraisal process.

Even with extraordinary efforts directed at behavioral monitoring and intervention, problems often occur, particularly with regard to assessing a physician's fitness to practice medicine. The term *fitness for duty*, borrowed from the military, is often applied when evaluating the rehabilitation of a provider accused of disruptive behavior. Finlayson et al. [7] described their 10-year experience analyzing data extracted from 381 physicians evaluated by the Vanderbilt Comprehensive Assessment Program from 2001 to 2012, 37.5 % of whom were referred to the program because of disruptive behavior. The authors found that after the release of the 2008 Joint Commission guidelines regarding behaviors that undermine a culture of safety [8], the number of physicians entering the program because of disruptive behavior increased. However, they also found that the disruptive physicians were less likely than others in the program to be considered unfit for practice. Among the physicians most likely to be judged "not fit to practice" were those referred for substance use (OR, 0.22; 95 % CI, 0.10–0.47; $P < 0.001$), mental health issues (OR, 0.14; 95 % CI, 0.06–0.31; $P < 0.001$), or sexual boundary issues (OR, 0.27; 95 % CI, 0.13–0.58; $P = 0.001$) (Table 16.11). The goal for all groups was to identify and intervene early for the best chance of good outcome.

TABLE 16.11. Likelihood of being judged "not fit to practice" among physicians referred for behavioral assessment [7].

Behavior	OR	95 % CI (P<0.001)
Sexual boundary issues	0.27	0.13–0.58
Substance use	0.22	0.10–0.47
Mental health issues	0.14	0.06–0.31
Disruptive behavior	Baseline	

Thus, it is important to realize that different degrees of impairment exist, and some categories of behavior—substance abuse and sexual boundary violations—need to be monitored very closely.

References

1. Kennedy MM. A crash course in conflict resolution. Physician Exec. 1998;24(4):60–1.
2. Pfifferling JH. The disruptive physician. A quality of professional life factor. Physician Exec. 1999;25(2):56–61.
3. Sotile WM, Sotile MO. Part 2, conflict management. How to shape positive relationships in medical practices and hospitals. Physician Exec. 1999;25(5):51–5.
4. Hills LS. 50 strategies for working well with doctors: a staff training tool. J Med Pract Manage. 2007;22(5):287–90.
5. Hickson GB, Pichert JW, Webb LE, Gabbe SG. A complimentary approach to promoting professionalism: identifying, measuring and addressing unprofessional behaviors. Acad Med. 2007;82(11):1040–8.
6. Holloway EL, Kusy M. Disruptive and toxic behaviors in healthcare: zero tolerance, the bottom line, and what to do about it. J Med Pract Manage. 2010;25(6):335–40.
7. Finlayson AJ, Dietrich MS, Neufeld R, Roback H, Martin PR. Restoring professionalism: the physician fitness-for-duty evaluation. Gen Hosp Psychiatry. 2013;35:659–63. doi:10.1016/j. genhosppsych.2013.06.009. pii:S0163-8343(13)00191-6.
8. The Joint Commission. Sentinel event alert: behaviors that undermine a culture of safety. 2008;(Issue 40). www.jointcommission. org/SentinelEvents/SentinelEventAlert/sea_40.htm. Accessed 20 Sept 2010.

Chapter 17
Educational Process

The basis of any educational process is to understand the learner as well as the lessons to be learned. It is clear that dealing with physicians requires an understanding of the uniqueness of the physician mindset. Doctors behave differently from other health-care staff in the areas of teamwork and negotiation. These differences require extra focus, as the ability to understand and leverage them into a more effective educational plan is crucial for the success of the program as well as the individual [1].

First, physicians are accustomed to making decisions autonomously, are quite competitive, and may find teamwork difficult at times. Second, however, they usually are skillful at negotiating complex issues with multiple parties. Although this trait typically is an advantage, occasionally extra negotiation is required to accomplish the task at hand. Third, their skills and coping mechanisms usually are firmly established after years of residency and fellowship training and often are resistant to change. Fourth, a physician's great ability to process, manage, and analyze information makes him or her an asset to the institution. Therefore, focusing or redirecting these skills in a positive way can facilitate the creation of common goals. Fifth, a physician's meticulous attention to detail occasionally may hamper discussions on quality of care and processes (Table 17.1). Because physician participation may

© Springer International Publishing Switzerland 2016   95
R.B. Vukmir, *Disruptive Healthcare Provider Behavior*,
DOI 10.1007/978-3-319-27924-4_17

TABLE 17.1. Physician traits making education challenging [1].

1. Autonomous decision-making
2. Complex negotiation skills
3. Established, ingrained skill sets
4. Ability to manage complex information streams
5. Meticulous attention to detail that may hamper discussions on quality of care and processes

TABLE 17.2. Guidelines for CME programs addressing disruptive behavior [2].

1. Know the audience before the presentation
2. Avoid potential pitfalls
3. Defuse defensiveness
4. Increase audience buy-in
5. Focus on theme
6. Use interactive teaching methods

be a great institutional asset, the best management approach is to educate physicians, solicit their input, and involve them in multidisciplinary quality initiatives and programs.

The advent of the new specialty-based maintenance of certification programs, with their emphasis on communication and professionalism, underscore the importance of nonclinical education. McLaren et al. [2] proposed several factors they feel are essential for an optimal continuing medical education (CME) program. First, for a program to be maximally effective, the presenters should know their audience and its expectations and goals (Table 17.2). Second, presenters should avoid pitfalls and potentially emotional issues early in the process, until team building is accomplished. Third, presenters should attempt to defuse any defensiveness on the part of the audience. Fourth, presenters should use techniques that capture the audience's attention and make it receptive to "buy-in." Fifth, the program should focus on positive themes, such as "rekindling of values" or "risk reduction," rather than using blame-assigning terminology. In summary, the successful interventional program uses interactive teaching methods to maximize audience participation and to foster self-awareness and reflection to achieve success.

Operating room nurses are often one of the best barometers of the acceptability of physician behavior. To improve the ability of perioperative nurses to address physician disruptive behavior, Saxton [3] studied the effects of a 2-day communication skill intervention program presented by a certified Crucial Conversations trainer. Among the 17 nurses who participated in the program, she found a significant improvement in mean self-efficacy scores immediately after the intervention as well as 4 weeks later. Most importantly, these nurses reported that after attending the program, they could manage disruptive physician behavior successfully most (71 %) of the time.

Disruptive behavior poses a particular challenge in academic medical centers, where the learning environment may be threatened. In this setting, disruptive physicians not only may cause staff conflict but also may be a poor role model for trainees, ultimately potentially placing patient safety at risk. Using a composite case study of an academic physician referred to a professional development program because of disruptive behavior, Samenow et al. [4] described how transformative learning concepts are used to design learning objectives, activities, and assessment tools for a curriculum to promote behavioral change in workplace interactions (Table 17.3). This intervention is based on a "safe group" process, whereby the physician's assumptions are critically analyzed, allowing exploration and development of new roles, skills, and coping behaviors. The effectiveness of this

TABLE 17.3. Transformative learning approach to disruptive behavior [4].

1. "Safe group" process examining physician's assumptions
2. Exercise to reflect and develop new roles and techniques
3. Timely feedback from colleagues, administrators, and institution
4. Successful return-to-practice program
5. Proactive approach toward medical intervention and prevention

TABLE 17.4. Elements of a real-time cultural change strategy [5].

1. Multistage approach
2. Phased in
3. Real-time
4. Systems based
5. Evidence based
6. Continuous evaluation

type of program relies on input and timely feedback to the physician from the institution, colleagues, and administrators. The goal is to return the physician to practice with more professional and effective behaviors.

Clearly, the best way to educate providers regarding professional conduct is to be proactive, by supporting programs aimed at preventing disruptive behavior, rather than reactive, by intervening after the behavior has occurred. According to Kusy and Holloway [5], the ability to achieve sustained real-time cultural change requires more than "just rolling out another educational program." They describe a "large-scale, real-time" permanent cultural change process founded on evidence-based research. Their approach focuses on several areas, including strategy formulation, change management, and service improvement. It stresses a multistep process that is phased in a real-time evidence-based, systems-oriented strategy that emphasizes continuous evaluation and reevaluation (Table 17.4). The ultimate goal is to achieve complete and sustained multidisciplinary organizational culture change through ongoing continuing professional education.

References

1. Van Dijck H. Hospital doctors behave differently, and only by respecting the fundamentals of professional organizations will managers be able to create common goals with professionals. Acta Clin Belg. 2014;69(4):309–11.

2. McLaren K, Lord J, Murray S. Perspective: delivering effective and engaging continuing medical education on physician's disruptive behavior. Acad Med. 2011;86(5):612–7.
3. Saxton R. Communication skills training to address disruptive physician behavior. AORN J. 2012;95(5):602–11.
4. Samenow CP, Worley LL, Neufeld R, Fishel T, Swiggart WH. Transformative learning in a professional development course aimed at addressing disruptive physician behavior: a composite case study. Acad Med. 2013;88(1):117–23.
5. Kusy M, Holloway EL. A field guide to real-time culture change: just "rolling out" a training program won't cut it. J Med Pract Manage. 2014;29(5):294–304.

Chapter 18
Management's Responsibility

Management of the health-care workplace in particular requires sustained administrative focus and support to shape positive relationships. According to Sotile and Sotile [1], "Managing workplace conflict is one of the most important, stressful, and time-consuming tasks faced by today's medical leaders." Although this comment seems to be describing contemporaneous events, ironically it was made in a 1999 article concerning health-care relationships. Since then, it has been recognized that poorly managed workplace conflicts may alienate patients, demoralize staff, increase employee turnover, and adversely affect referral relationships and third-party insurers focused on customer satisfaction (Table 18.1).

Health-care executives cannot solve this problem simply by improving their conflict management skills or by policing offenders. Disruptive behavior does not occur in a vacuum; therefore, it is important for it to be interpreted in the wider context of individual and system performance. Often, the behavior provides a clue to the existence of underlying individual or systemic problems in the medical care process. True leadership, then, requires intervention aimed at fostering a culture of healthy interpersonal dynamics: the key is to think,

© Springer International Publishing Switzerland 2016   101
R.B. Vukmir, *Disruptive Healthcare Provider Behavior*,
DOI 10.1007/978-3-319-27924-4_18

TABLE 18.1. Effects of workplace conflict [1].

1. Alienation of patients
2. Staff demoralization
3. Increased staff turnover
4. Damage to referral relationships
5. Impact on third-party insurers
6. Decreased patient satisfaction

TABLE 18.2. Steps to shaping positive health-care relationships [1].

1. Realize that problems cannot be solved by self-improvement or policing alone
2. Address larger contextual issues
3. Examine for actual patient care issues
4. Foster a positive interpersonal culture dynamic
5. Think and intervene systematically

analyze, and intervene systemically (Table 18.2). Moreover, a good ethical culture starts at the top of the organization, with no double standard for administration versus employees. Physician leaders must set the tone for an ethical and honest workplace for all health-care providers.

As Ward [2] pointed out, the success of any business enterprise is determined by the employees and their work performance. She suggested that the acceptance of disruptive behavior, such as verbal abuse, based on the institutional status of the perpetrator demonstrates bad management. On the other hand, the hallmarks of good management include well-written policies, physician champions, strong executive leadership, and the willingness of managers to try new approaches to help the staff develop more robust skill sets to achieve and maintain a healthier work environment (Table 18.3).

Clearly, medical executives should spend more time inspiring great employees and building productive teams and less time managing disruptive behavior (Table 18.4) [3]. To that end, the goal is to reduce the frequency and intensity of aberrant behavior so that more time may be dedicated to more productive, integrative activities. Therefore, the physician

TABLE 18.3. Attributes of good management [2].

1. Well-written policies
2. Physician champions
3. Strong executives
4. Willingness to try novel approaches

TABLE 18.4. Leadership goals in dealing with disruptive behavior [3].

1. Inspire employees and build productive teams
2. Diminish the frequency and intensity of disruptive behavior
3. Identify roles, rights, and responsibilities
4. Define the chain of accountability

leader should identify his or her role, rights, responsibilities, and ultimate accountability in addressing these concerns.

Disruptive behavior by physicians places a heavy burden on medical groups, yet practice leaders and administrators often lack the tools to address it, or they may simply ignore the behavior because the misbehaving physician brings much revenue to the practice [4]. This phenomenon is more likely to occur when the practice manager is employed by the group rather than being outside the administrative chain.

Every institution should consider the use of consultants to recommend ways to foster a respectful work environment. These professionals bring many contributions to the table, including outside expertise and authority. However, these arrangements must be tempered by a cost analysis. Moreover, a consultant may have less understanding of local relationships and sensitivities.

If there is a delay in dealing with a physician's misconduct, he or she may continue to act out, in ways that would not be tolerated in other staff members. Although significant focus has been directed on serious behavioral issues such as impairment or addiction, more indolent issues often have been overlooked or allowed to continue unabated. Bauman [4] suggested ways to recognize and manage less extreme behaviors such as professional misconduct. In his article "Disruptive Physicians…

and How to Deal with Them," he offers comprehensive tools to identify disruptive behavior, as well as "do and don't" lists and a simple test to provide an unbiased assessment of what steps need to be taken to manage the problem.

As pointed out by Youssi [5], the Joint Commission for Accreditation of Healthcare Organizations (JCAHO) empowers a facility's medical executive committee to act on the staff's behalf to bring recommendations to the governing body concerning physician disruptive behavior. The medical executive committee is accountable for recommending, for the governing body's approval, six pivotal actions to help identify and address the physician with disruptive behavior (Table 18.5): (1) establish mechanisms and explicit criteria for reviewing credentials for medical staff applicants; (2) consider individuals for medical staff membership who can be part of the solution; (3) define and delineate medical staff privileges as well as criteria for reward or removal; (4) ensure medical staff participation in any process improvement initiatives for maximal chance of success; (5) establish a procedure to restrict or terminate medical staff membership if remediation fails; and (6) establish a fair and transparent process to hear and evaluate disagreements that may arise during the resolution phase.

To address the question postulated by Pearson and Porath [6]—"What is a leader to do when managing incivility in the health care workplace?"—the authors offered a nine-point action plan to assist in managing disruptive behavior (Table 18.6). First, it is important to set a zero-tolerance policy for all staff working in the health-care arena. Second, self-reflection is a crucial part of the process; therefore, each leader should take an honest look in the mirror. Third, trou-

TABLE 18.5. Six pivotal actions by a medical executive committee [5].

1. Establish mechanisms and criteria for reviewing credentials
2. Consider individuals for medical staff membership
3. Delineate clinical privileges
4. Ensure participation in the medical staff improvement process
5. Establish procedure for medical staff termination
6. Create a fair and equitable hearing process

TABLE 18.6. Steps for leaders to manage incivility [6].

1. Establish zero-tolerance expectations
2. Take an honest look in the mirror
3. Weed out trouble before it starts
4. Embrace and teach civility
5. Always keep an ear to the ground and listen carefully
6. When incivility occurs, quash it immediately
7. Monitor and heed warning signals
8. Don't give a pass to the big fish
9. Invest in the post-departure interview

ble should be anticipated and thwarted before it takes hold within the organization so that a lengthy extraction process is avoided. Fourth, civility should be the cornerstone of the organization's ethos and should be taught to all staff, embraced by administration, and integrated in all procedures and programs. Fifth, the leader should remain vigilant and aware of environmental clues so he or she can intervene early and proactively, which is a much more desirable pathway than a cleanup process after an event occurs. Sixth, if and when incivility occurs, it must be dealt with quickly and decisively to keep the worrisome behavior from cross-contaminating the staff further. Seventh, early warning signals of unrest, whether inside or outside the program, should be heeded; rumors of a problem often are correct in cases such as these. Eighth, excuses must not be made for disruptive physicians who are powerful, well-placed, and/or significant financial contributors to the medical center. This indeed is the most critical point for most institutions. Whenever a pass is given to an administrator, the physician with the most hospital admissions, the surgeon performing the most operations, or the investigator receiving the most research funding, the program is sure to fail. Ninth, perhaps one of the most valuable assets is the exit interview for staff members who leave the institution. It can provide incredibly valuable information concerning problems within the organization. Often, a significant amount of money is paid to consultants to analyze deficiencies and sometimes to reinvent the wheel; however, employees who choose to leave the institution, especially those who are disgruntled, often have much better insight into areas that need improvement.

Recently, the Joint Commission's Leadership Blog summarized several groups' recommendations for addressing disruptive behaviors (Table 18.7) [7–9]. First, make behavioral expectations explicit by defining them in a code of conduct supported by appropriate policies. Second, ensure that the board of directors gives robust support to the administration and clinical leaders during program implementation. Third, provide education, support, and training to those dealing with disruptive and intimidating behavior. Fourth, screen for stressors, particularly health and personal issues, among all providers involved. It should be clear by now that this phenomenon involves all health-care providers and personnel involved in the care delivery system. Fifth, establish proactive surveillance systems to document and record events specific to this process. Sixth, deal with infringements and violations in a manner that is both consistent and transparent to observers. Seventh, deal with lower-level aberrant behavior early in the process to prevent a more significant problem down the road. Small but persistent problems often turn into larger, more significant ones. Eighth, provide a system of graduated responses—

TABLE 18.7. Joint Commission's summary of recommendations [7–9].

1. Establish a code of conduct supported by appropriate policies to explicitly define expectations
2. Ensure support of clinicians by board of directors during the implementation phase
3. Provide training and support for those experiencing the behavior
4. Screen all involved parties for personal and health issues
5. Establish proactive surveillance programs
6. Deal consistently and transparently with transgressions
7. Confront low-level aberrant behaviors at the beginning
8. Establish a graduated series of responses—informal, formal, disciplinary, regulatory—based on incident severity
9. Provide resources to those involved in and affected by the disruptive behavior

informal, formal, disciplinary, and regulatory—according to incident severity, which will allow the proper match of resources to the intervention. Ninth, ensure sufficient resources to help those responsible for as well as those affected by the intimidating behavior. The key is to define goals and expectations from the start for health-care providers.

Solutions are not set in stone and should be reviewed, and potentially revised, as new information and techniques become available. The American Board of Internal Medicine (ABIM), American College of Physicians (ACP)/American Society of Internal Medicine (ASIM), and the European Federation of Internal Medicine (ESIM) issued a consortium statement defining several rationales and commitments with the goal of maintaining medical professionalism [10]. The fundamental principles are primacy of patient welfare, patient autonomy, and social justice (Table 18.8). The consortium also defined ten professional responsibilities necessary for a successful clinical practice (Table 18.9): (1) a demonstrated

TABLE 18.8. Charter on professionalism: fundamental principles [10].

1. Primacy of patient welfare
2. Patient autonomy
3. Social justice

TABLE 18.9. Charter on professionalism: professional responsibilities [10].

1. Professional competence
2. Honesty with patients
3. Patient confidentiality
4. Maintenance of appropriate relationships with patients
5. Improvement in quality of care
6. Improvement in access to care
7. Just distribution of finite resources
8. Scientific knowledge
9. Maintenance of trust by managing conflicts of interests
10. Professional responsibilities

commitment to professional competence, (2) complete honesty in patient dealings, (3) patient confidentiality, (4) an ongoing commitment to maintaining appropriate relations with patients, (5) continual efforts to improve the quality of patient care, (6) a commitment to improving access to care, (7) a just and fair distribution of finite care resources, (8) care decisions founded on scientific knowledge, (9) maintenance of trust by managing real or potential conflicts of interest, and (10) a commitment to maintain one's professional responsibilities.

Rosenstein and O'Daniel [11] surveyed more than 100 hospitals to evaluate the effects of disruptive behaviors on communication and collaboration among medical staff as well as their impact on patient care. Based on their findings, the authors offered ten recommendations for managing these behaviors (Table 18.10). (1) The institution's staff must recognize the problem and be aware of its scope. This is best achieved by distributing a confidential self-assessment survey to personnel asking them to report on behaviors or events that have had a negative impact on their work or on patient care. (2) To achieve success, the entire staff must be committed to cultural change; therefore, the organization should adopt a "top-down, bottom-up" approach in which all parties, management, and workers are responsible for their behavior and are expected to adhere to a clearly defined code of conduct.

TABLE 18.10. Recommendations for managing disruptive behavior [11].

1. Recognition and awareness
2. Cultural commitment, leadership, champions
3. Policies and procedures
4. Incident reporting
5. Structure and process
6. Initiating factors
7. Education and training
8. Communication tools
9. Discussion forums
10. Intervention strategies

Support by staff from throughout the organization acting as champions for the cause will facilitate this transition. (3) The organization must develop clear policies, procedures, and guidelines that set forth a zero-tolerance approach toward those who are not in compliance. (4) The organization should have a standardized incident-reporting process to avoid the vagaries of many informal reports. (5) A consistent, uniform method should be in place for addressing the issues. (6) A better understanding of the initiating factors and high-risk scenarios is needed to avoid conflict in the first place. (7) Comprehensive training and education should be provided to all staff. (8) Efforts should be made to improve communication skills among the majority of the staff instead of focusing resources on a few high-risk providers. (9) Discussion forums, group meetings, and other programs should be developed to encourage staff interaction. (10) Intervention strategies should be implemented to lessen the impact of disruptive events. For example, some facilities have a formalized policy (e.g., "condition D," "code white," "code pink") in which coworkers or designated individuals are summoned to a disruptive event to serve as witnesses or mediators. Strength in numbers creates an environment in which workers are more likely to speak out and begin the process to effect change.

In summary, the overall goal is an individualized program that takes into account facility nuances to ensure the greatest success at each institution.

References

1. Sotile WM, Sotile MO. How to shape positive relationships in medical practices and hospitals. Physician Exec. 1999;25(4):57–61.
2. Ward S. What you as a manager can do to overcome verbal abuse of staff. OR Manager. 2002;18(12):1, 12–5.
3. Keogh T, Martin W. Managing unmanageable physicians: leadership, stewardship and disruptive behavior. Physician Exec. 2004;30(5):18–22.
4. Bauman RR. Disruptive physicians…and how to deal with them. J Med Pract Manage. 2006;22(2):79–83.

5. Youssi MD. JCAHO standards help address disruptive physician behavior—doctors, nurses and disruptive behavior—Joint Commission for accreditation of healthcare organizations standards. Physician Exec. 2002; Nov–Dec:47–8.

6. Pearson CM, Porath CL. On the nature, consequences and remedies of workplace incivility: no time for "nice"? Think again. Acad Manage Exec. 2005;19(1):7–18.

7. Swiggart WH, Dewey CM, Hickson GB, Finlayson AJ, Spickard WA. A plan for identification, treatment and remediation of disruptive behaviors in physicians. Front Health Serv Manage. 2009;25(4):3–11.

8. Hills LS. 50 strategies for working well with doctors: a staff training tool. J Med Pract Manage. 2007;22(5):287–90.

9. Wyatt RM. Revisiting disruptive and inappropriate behavior: five years after standards introduced. Jt Comm Physician Blog. 2014; Oct 02:1–3.

10. ABIM Foundation, ACP-ASIM Foundation, European Federation of Internal Medicine. Medical professionalism in a new millennium: a physician charter. Ann Intern Med. 2002; 136:243–6.

11. Rosenstein AH, O'Daniel M. A survey of the impact of disruptive behaviors and communication defects on patient safety. Jt Comm J Qual Patient Saf. 2008;34(8):464–71.

Chapter 19
Conclusion

Disruptive physician behavior is not a new phenomenon; it has been described since the beginning of the twentieth century. Its negative consequences on the reputation of the health-care field, staff morale, finances, and quality of care are now well recognized. Although much of today's discussion regarding professional misconduct focuses only on physicians, some experts have recognized a more nuanced scenario involving nursing, paraprofessional, and administrative personnel.

The scope of the problem suggests that great strides have been made in addressing training, certification, and civil and even criminal transgressions related to disruptive behavior. However, attempts to confront the more subtle but no less worrisome adverse effects of disruptive behavior on the health-care delivery system have been less successful. Many of these efforts have focused on the credentialing and privileging process and have been effective only in select cases.

An organization-wide approach offers the best chance of success in addressing the complicated area of disruptive behavior. This strategy begins with recommendations by professional specialty societies, licensing boards, and regional medical societies; the Joint Commission and state boards of health, for example, have provided clear mandates addressing the issue of disruptive behavior. Finally, site-based intervention should be driven by the facility's bylaws, clear pathways for education and remediation, and processes and procedures. Informal, after-the-fact intervention carries much less validity with the staff.

© Springer International Publishing Switzerland 2016   111
R.B. Vukmir, *Disruptive Healthcare Provider Behavior*,
DOI 10.1007/978-3-319-27924-4_19

TABLE 19.1. Maturation of the analysis.

1. Quandary: person or situation?
2. Involvement of physicians, nurses, and administration
3. Change in focus from provider to patient safety impact
4. Interaction of situation and all providers involved
5. Incorporation of impact on patient care

The analysis of disruptive behavior has certainly matured over time (Table 19.1). First, there has been a quandary regarding whether the person or the situation is the problem that needs to be resolved, with passionate proponents of each theory. Second, it is now well established that the problem is at least as common in nursing, with a renewed focus on hospital administration as a nidus as well. Third, focus also has shifted from provider impact to patient safety goals in the consideration of disruptive behavior. Fourth, it now is understood that the provider is not the only component; the encounter and the interaction of all parties are equally important. Lastly, patients now are recognized as sometimes contributing to the difficult encounter milieu.

Profiling the disruptive behavior offers additional insight into the likelihood of improvement (Table 19.2). The key is to define the behavior prospectively in objective terms that can be measured and analyzed easily. Disruptive behaviors range from overt "acting out" to more subtle, less obvious conduct. It is important to avoid imposing labels, personalizing the analysis, and using conflicted or biased sources of information. The term *disruptive* should not be used inappropriately to label well-intentioned criticism of the system or its processes, which may be warranted. The appearance of bias will cause the system to lose all credibility.

Some units in the facility, as well as some specialty practices, may warrant extra surveillance and intervention. These areas are more prone to stress and tend to be associated with high-risk disease, highly complex cases, unpredictable flow and needs, and multiple providers with conflicting care priorities;

TABLE 19.2. Analysis of the behavior.

1. Define the behavior in objective terms
2. Monitor the entire behavior spectrum
3. Avoid imposing labels
4. Avoid personalizing the analysis
5. Avoid biased information sources
6. Avoid inappropriate labeling of quality concerns

TABLE 19.3. High-risk location and specialty profile for disruptive behavior.

1. High-risk disease states
2. Highly complex decision-making
3. Unpredictable flow and demands
4. Presence of multiple providers
5. Conflicting care priorities
6. Scarcity of resources
7. Little capability to adjust staffing
8. Interface of flexible–inflexible units
9. Staffing ratio limitations
10. Little employee control or input

they also are under-resourced with little adjustment capability and have inflexible interfaces and staffing ratios with little employee input or control (Table 19.3). The last point is most important, as personnel function better in an environment in which they have some control. The high-risk areas include the operating suite, labor and delivery area, intensive care unit, and emergency department (Table 19.4). With regard to specialty areas at greater risk for disruptive behavior, the surgical specialties are overrepresented, including general surgery, cardiothoracic surgery, neurosurgery, orthopedics, and obstetric/gynecologic surgery (Table 19.5).

Perhaps the greatest impact on reducing the risk of disruptive behavior may be derived from starting early in the process by teaching professional accountability at the medical school and residency levels. It is recognized that long-term practice patterns are established early in the educational

TABLE 19.4. High-risk hospital areas.

1. Operating room
2. Labor and delivery area
3. Intensive care unit
4. Emergency department

TABLE 19.5. High-risk specialties.

1. General surgery
2. Cardiothoracic surgery
3. Neurosurgery
4. Orthopedics
5. Obstetrics/gynecology

process; therefore, behaviors physicians witness during their training likely will dictate their own behavior when they subsequently are in practice.

Even the most sophisticated facilities, those that perform comprehensive system analyses, eventually look to the individual when seeking an etiology for bad behavior rather than evaluating the entire system. The psychological dynamics often are complicated by numerous theories implicated in the analysis, many of which attempt to classify a personality type or types associated with disruptive behavior. Efforts also have been made to determine whether the behavior is associated with stress, illness, or conflict dynamics.

Often, the nursing interface provides another crucible for conflict in this arena. Early studies suggested that nurses experience disruptive behavior more frequently than physicians, whereas later studies indicated that both professions experience it in equal measure. Another, perhaps underappreciated, area of conflict involves nurse-to-nurse interactions.

As always, analyses into disruptive behavior are focused on patient safety, as well as the individual's well-being. Although there is an inherent association between disruptive behavior and adverse outcomes, proving a link to causality has been rather difficult.

The basis of any successful interventional program is the institution of specific policies or guidelines that, ideally, are based on benchmarks of an organized group, such as the Joint Commission or a state medical society. These programs work best when all parties buy in to and support them. Most importantly, top-down support is needed from the administration for the program to be accepted throughout the organization.

Whereas disruptive behavior is obviously a detriment to staff, the economic harm it causes may be more nuanced, although it certainly is tangible. Its effects on the cost side manifest as increased employee turnover and retraining, loss of productivity, and decreased efficiency. The revenue side is affected by patient loss, a decreased influx of new patients, adverse impacts on the service line, financial penalties, and loss of external incentives, the last of which is the subject of legal controversy. Disruptive behavior events may trigger many regulatory, statutory, and litigation influences. Several outside agencies have established guidelines mandating that disruptive behavior be confronted and remedied, leaving the facility no choice but to address the issue.

Strategies for improving a disruptive work environment typically require a multifaceted, multidisciplinary approach. Various groups have offered problem–solution, list-oriented methods for dealing the dilemma. Although many of these approaches have proven successful at some locations, they should be tailored and adapted to the individual site.

The cornerstone of any quality improvement program is education, including the training of new staff members as well as continuing education for established practitioners. These interventions, however, are applied differently at academic versus clinical health-care centers.

Dealing with disruptive physician behavior may be the most time-consuming task for hospital administrators, distracting them from more mainstream and productive endeavors. As stated previously, their participation in and support of programs to address toxic behavior and ensure a civil working environment are essential. The system must work for all parties—nurses, physicians, and administrative personnel—for enduring success.

Appendix: Situational Analysis and Approach to Case Scenarios

These scenarios are offered as illustrative examples of potential behavioral issues and are not portrayals of actual provider encounters.

Case 1: "Always Unavailable" (Physician Is Never Available for Call Responsibilities)

Situation

The concerns were the same. He seemed to never answer any paging calls or service requests from the hospital staff. This behavior was noted by almost all staff, including the unit secretaries, nurses, and other physicians. The nurses were especially worried, because at night they felt patient care suffered when he took so long to respond.

At one point, another employee overheard him in the elevator joking that if it were "really important," they would call him back. "If they call once, it probably wasn't important. The second time, I might pay attention; the third time, it is usually something, so I answer, because it is important." He chuckled again to a colleague as they exited the elevator and was overheard by patients, visitors, and other staff members.

The physician had been on staff at the institution for a long time and universally was considered a good physician. He was

© Springer International Publishing Switzerland 2016   117
R.B. Vukmir, *Disruptive Healthcare Provider Behavior*,
DOI 10.1007/978-3-319-27924-4

intelligent and technically proficient, and others felt that he had a nice bedside manner.

The physician's lack of on-call availability was discussed with him previously by a medical staff officer. At that time, he shrugged off the concern, reiterating his belief that "if it is important, they will call me back." The officer recommended that he updates his technologic capability by using a smartphone rather than his paging system. This would allow him to be more readily available to the nurses as well as to other health-care professionals that might need his services. He responded that he had started his career with a paging system, and that is how he would end it as well, saying, "People will call me all the time if I get one of those damn cell phones."

Recently, the problem came up again when he was needed for a patient issue and waited an hour to return the call. The floor nursing staff eventually decided to call a rapid response event rather than wait any longer. The patient was transferred to a critical care unit, but no associated adverse events occurred. The next day, the chief nursing officer filed a formal complaint concerning the doctor's chronic call unavailability behavior.

Issue

When a doctor is on call for unassigned patients, he or she is expected to return calls within a maximum of 30 min. Although the physician is not required to appear for care, he or she should respond to the call to enact a care plan. This time frame is extrapolated to the same parameter for calls concerning the physician's own patients or those of his or her call group.

Approach

1. Every step should be taken to ensure that the provider has an effective individualized communication system (Table A.1).

2. It should be determined whether the call schedule is reasonable and accepted by the physicians in that call group.
3. At the first sign of this type of behavior, informal peer-to-peer mediation should occur.
4. The initial intervention should always be face to face.
5. This meeting should be followed by a formal medical staff intervention, initially involving the department chair, to define expectations.
6. If further intervention is needed, it may require the involvement of the vice president of medical affairs (VPMA), the chief medical officer (CMO), or the medical staff president.
7. The behavior should be tracked, monitored, and benchmarked at that facility if intervention is required.
8. If informal approaches have been unsuccessful, a formal action plan should be formulated, implemented, and monitored. This plan may involve temporary suspension of admitting privileges.
9. Further infractions may involve loss of staff privileges and may trigger a mandatory report to the National Practitioner Database (NPDB) or other regulatory agencies.

TABLE A.1. Steps in mediating delayed on-call response behavior.

1. Ensure an effective communication system
2. Establish an acceptable, equitable call system
3. Begin with informal peer-to-peer mediation
4. Then hold a face-to-face meeting
5. Continue with formal mediation with the department chair
6. Follow with the VPMA, CMO, or medical staff president
7. Track, monitor, and benchmark the intervention
8. Take formal action by restricting admission privileges
9. Submit report to external databank if required

Case 2: "Bad Day" (Physician Has Violent Outbursts in the Workplace)

Situation

The word spread through the hospital quickly. He was having a really bad day. His operating suite had to be changed because of a problem with the room. There was an anesthesia delay because of decreased staff availability. The final straw came when the robotic arm he needed for his 9 am surgical procedure broke. The nurses were overheard at the front desk stating, "He is going to blow a gasket now."

They were indeed correct, as the scenario had repeated itself many times before. When he found out about the broken robotic arm, he began to scream and curse in the anesthesia preoperative staging area. This diatribe was overheard by staff, patients, and families. One of the anesthesiologists, with whom he is friends, was summoned to de-escalate the situation.

Although the content of his outburst was valid, his coworkers felt his method of delivery was not helpful to them. There was no debate regarding the inappropriateness of the setting, where the comments were made, or the public discussion of work circumstances. The staff felt that the surgeon's grievances should have been directed at the administration and not them; they were simply trying their best to move patients through the operating room (OR) under difficult circumstances. Interestingly, the staff agreed with his sentiments; there had been recent staffing cuts and equipment unavailability.

The surgeon cooled down and started his next case. The remainder of the day went on uneventfully. The next day, the patient advocate received a complaint from a family member concerning the behavior exhibited in the OR.

Issue

Problems occur every day in medicine; the key is to navigate through them efficiently and effectively. It is clear that discussing difficult issues such as these in public is neither appropriate nor effective in their resolution. Members of the public should not be exposed to work-related discussions. Likewise, solutions to problems such as these typically are not achieved in this type of open-air forum.

Approach

1. The first step is isolation of the controversy (Table A.2). Every attempt should be made to protect the other health-care workers, as well as patients and their family members, from being exposed to this discussion in the public realm.
2. Once the disruption has been isolated, a formal debriefing of all involved parties must be performed.
3. The provider exhibiting the behavior should undergo immediate counseling, with an emphasis on anger management. The nature of this transgression requires its immediate correction, and intervention must go beyond a simple informal, collegial discussion.
4. A formal intervention process must be initiated, with its components tailored to the incident's severity.
5. The intervention should begin with a peer group analysis, including multidisciplinary input, which often facilitates better understanding and self-awareness, providing a wider perspective into the behavior and offering a more balanced insight.
6. The results of this analysis should be submitted to the medical staff officer for recommendations based on the facility's bylaws.
7. However, any recommendations, guidance, or penalties must come from a professional peer group pathway.
8. The intervention should have full administrative support and sufficient resources to carry it out.
9. External referral for forensic psychiatric evaluation may be necessary.
10. It should be noted that these cases are especially difficult, because they often involve providers who have concentrated

power and influence based on financial contributions to the institution. These physicians may be responsible for a large proportion of the hospital's admissions or may otherwise contribute significantly to the hospital census. Likewise, specialists or surgeons who contribute disproportionately to the procedural product of the facility also may figure prominently in these cases.

11. An effective administrator recognizes that there must be no appearance of impropriety or favoritism and incidents must not be treated differently based on economic factors, hierarchical status, or job role.

12. At the same time, it is essential to realize that there may be operational issues related to equipment, staffing, or expertise that are unveiled in times of stress.

13. Self-assertiveness training for the staff would be helpful in restoring balance to the unit.

TABLE A.2. Steps in dealing with inappropriate verbal behavior.

1. Isolate the controversy
2. Conduct a formal debriefing with all parties
3. Offer immediate formal counseling stressing anger management techniques
4. Initiate a formal individualized intervention process
5. Conduct a peer group evaluation
6. Seek multidisciplinary input to provide a balanced perspective
7. Follow professional peer group recommendations
8. Obtain full administrative support
9. Refer the provider to a forensic psychiatrist
10. Ensure universal standards for all staff regardless of their financial contribution
11. Monitor for favoritism
12. Ensure no operational, equipment, or staffing issues exist
13. Offer self-assertiveness training for staff

Case 3: "At It Again" (Physician Has Sexual Boundary Issues)

Situation

The atmosphere of the unit was pretty loose at times, and there was a lot of joking and sexual innuendo among the staff. The unit provided emergency, high-risk critical care, and the staff used this as a rationale for this aberrant behavior. This behavior was pervasive, took several different forms, and involved and/or affected many staff members. The teasing was ubiquitous, and some employees, both male and female, expressed concerns about it. Some felt it was doctors targeting nurses, whereas others witnessed nurses participating in the joking as well.

The exploits of one of the unit's physicians were well known throughout the institution. He had had several marriages, divorces, and subsequent relationships. He seemed to take a particular interest in one of the nurses, speaking to her and touching her in a manner that seemed inappropriate for the workplace. However, some staff noted a reciprocal relationship, with both parties actively involved in this behavior. Nonetheless, the situation made some workers on the unit uncomfortable, and some complained about it.

The rumor was that this doctor and this nurse had been involved in a relationship for the past 6 months. However, some staff members believed that their clandestine relationship had ended abruptly. There also was talk that he and the nurse had exchanged risqué photographs and text messages. Despite the various theories regarding what happened and who had ended the relationship though, the physician somehow seemed to always be at the center of this aberrant behavior.

Eventually, the nurse filed a sexual harassment complaint against the physician. His initial response was that her report was a retaliatory move because he had just ended their relationship. His response to the investigative committee was that "she did not seem to mind when we were in a relationship, only after I broke it off." The nursing administrator also took part in the investigation, and when she interviewed the nurse about her complaint, the nurse admitted that she indeed had had an at-work relationship with the physician, but as his behavior became more inappropriate, she ended the relationship.

Issue

Every facility has the obligation to ensure a workplace free from any verbal or physical harassment that may be construed as establishing or perpetuating an environment in which customary sexual boundaries are violated.

Approach

Many excuses and rationalizations often are presented for why things are "just that way" at a particular institution. This behavior tends to be concentrated in high-risk, high-acuity units, such as the OR, intensive care unit (ICU), and emergency department (ED). In these areas, the stakes are perceived to be high; therefore, the behaviors exhibited there may be extreme as well.

1. No excuses should be given based on the acuity, work requirements, or productivity of the unit (Table A.3).
2. Guidelines on proper sexual boundaries in the workplace should be documented and regularly updated.
3. These guidelines should be accessible to all employees in an electronic, easily updatable format.
4. A confidential multidisciplinary investigation should be initiated, with all involved parties participating in the interview process.
5. The involved parties should be separated or chaperoned in the workplace until the investigation has been completed satisfactorily.
6. Parties identified as having committed a transgression should have their privileging status evaluated according to the medical staff bylaws.

7. Consultation with the hospital's legal counsel is necessary in all scenarios such as these but especially important in this one.
8. The remediation plan may include reeducation, practice restriction, or revocation of staff privileges.
9. Consultation with law enforcement may be required in egregious cases in which summary suspension will occur.
10. Referral to an outside reeducation program on sexual boundaries usually is required, as these cases typically are associated with a high recidivism rate. These programs range from continuing medical education symposiums to in-depth forensic psychiatric assessments including a diagnosis and fitness-for-duty recommendation.
11. Ongoing education of staff on how to identify, report, and prevent sexual boundary violations is a crucial part of the process in both the present and the future.
12. Sensitivity and impulse control training may be effective in these cases.

TABLE A.3. Keys to handling sexual boundary issues.

1. Set uniform standards for all providers independent of their workload or productivity
2. Document guidelines and update them regularly
3. Make sure these guidelines are easily accessible, ideally in an electronic format
4. Conduct a confidential multidisciplinary interview of all involved parties
5. Separate or chaperone involved parties until they are exonerated
6. Evaluate the privileges of transgressors according to bylaws
7. Consult hospital legal counsel
8. Develop and execute a remediation plan that includes reeducation, practice restriction, or privilege revocation
9. Consult law enforcement if necessary
10. Refer the provider to an external sexual boundary reeducation program
11. Provide ongoing reeducation of staff
12. Recommend sensitivity and impulse control training

Case 4: "Not Taking That Order" (Nurse Refuses to Complete Proper Order)

Situation

She was an experienced nurse with a tough, resilient exterior who was widely known as a great patient care advocate. She was passionate about the nursing profession and her role in it. She was a stickler for detail and always went above and beyond the basic knowledge required to administer medications. She was especially interested in the drugs used in the critical care unit, noting various dosing strategies, side effects, and possible drug interactions, and she served as the nursing representative on the hospital-based pharmacology and therapeutics committee.

It was well-known at the hospital that she commonly refused resident physicians' orders when she felt there was uncertainty, inaccuracy, or outright error involved. Although the site used a computerized physician order entry (CPOE) system, incompatibilities and errors occasionally occurred.

That night she was working in the neurologic trauma ICU. A patient was brought in who had suffered an abdominal gunshot wound, and he was admitted to the unit after an exploratory laparotomy. The patient was still hypotensive after a massive volume resuscitation of crystalloid, colloid, and blood. His central venous pressure (CVP) catheter was dysfunctional and had to be removed.

The surgical resident was writing orders and requested the addition of intravenous norepinephrine, a direct-acting sympathetic alpha-1 and beta-1 adrenergic agonist, at a dose of 1 μg/kg/min. The nurse suggested that he consider another intervention, and her rationale was sound. First, the dose was a little high for initiation of therapy. Second, she thought a CVP line should be reestablished to gauge the patient's volume status, as he might still have been hypovolemic. Finally, the patient was on phenelzine, an older mono-amine oxidase inhibitor antidepressant that may cross-react with direct-acting amine-based vasopressors such as norepinephrine.

After this discussion between the resident and the nurse, the resident consulted with the senior resident, who asked him to put the nurse on the phone. The senior resident asked the nurse if she was refusing to implement the resident's order. The nurse stated that yes, she was, and that she wasn't "going to hang that med for him or anyone else." She then said, "Why don't you talk to your attending, or critical care, or someone else who knows what the hell they are doing?" The senior resident responded, "I am the doctor, and you are the nurse. I write the orders, and you follow them; that's how it goes."

The nurse was summoned to the director's office, where she was told the incident had been reported to the nursing administration to be evaluated as an episode of disruptive provider behavior cited by the physician.

Issue

From a critical care perspective, all the issues raised by the nurse indeed were correct and should have warranted reconsideration by both parties involved.

Approach

These cases often are problematic, with battle lines drawn quickly between nurses and physicians (Table A.4).

1. The approach should focus first on the actual behavior rather than a proxy battle between physicians and nurses.
2. An analysis should be undertaken by a multidisciplinary working group, including both nurses and physicians, to avoid the appearance of favoritism.

3. In factual disputes, such as the one in this scenario, an expert panel must be involved.
4. Although one or both parties may be correct in their assessment, the behavior involved should be addressed.
5. Informal mediation, with both parties involved, is a good solution for the initial back-and-forth communication.
6. Education of all staff is critically important so that everyone learns to appreciate one another's roles and responsibilities.
7. A multidisciplinary task force meeting may help address issues of concern to both nursing and physician services.
8. In cases such as this, behavioral counseling often is effective.
9. Training staff in negotiation skills often helps resolve common operational disputes, such as the one in this scenario.

TABLE A.4. Handling nurse–physician interaction problems.

1. Focus on the specific behavior, not proxy a battle
2. Conduct a multidisciplinary analysis including nurses and physicians
3. Convene an expert panel for factual issues
4. Focus on the behavior, not on who is right
5. Initiate informal mediation
6. Educate all staff
7. Assemble a multidisciplinary operational task force
8. Use a behavioral counseling approach
9. Offer training in negotiation skills for operational issues

Case 5: "There Goes Another One" (Administrator Responsible for Employee Turnover)

Situation

The facility had always been known as a tough place to work, with an extremely high employee turnover rate for the area. Despite the hard work and high volumes though, other factors seemed to be involved in the staffing problem. Based on murmurings by the hospital's workers, an administrative team they perceived as tough was thought to be one of the main causes for the overall job dissatisfaction.

Employee turnover occurred at both the service-line managerial and staff levels. These losses were extremely costly to the institution, with focus diverted from institutional goals and objectives. In addition, the expenses incurred by the facility in orienting and training so many new employees were significant.

During an evaluation by a group of outside experts, one of the reviewers noted a lack of diversity in the facility's workforce. Most well-respected institutions have a multigenerational workforce; however, the high turnover rate at this hospital had resulted in a one-dimensional employee pool. The evaluators commented that this homogeneity deprives newer employees from benefiting from the on-the-job experience passed on by older workers.

Moreover, some employees overheard administrative staff publicly making comments they felt were inappropriate. Although the administrators typically couched these statements in financial terms related to institutional goals and objectives, which is acceptable and, in some cases, desirable as a management tool, many of their comments were related to the physical stamina, appearance, and training of the staff.

Also, employees overheard administrators complaining about employee salaries, on-the-job injury statistics, and education costs for the workforce.

At a board of directors meeting, some of these issues were discussed, and a request was made to address the concerns of the external review agency.

Issue

Although a need exists for proactive institutional management, one must keep in mind that presentation is key. Another important point to consider is that disruptive behavior may involve any member of the health-care team, not just physicians and nurses. Administrators are under constant pressure to demonstrate financial accountability, both internally and to the external marketplace.

Approach

1. The key to successful institutional change and progress is to obtain employee buy-in. Workers who are sold on the ideology will help everyone succeed in patient care goals (Table A.5).
2. Employees are most likely to give their support if they feel they have a say in the change process, meaning real representation and a voice in planning sessions.
3. The staff should be polled for their opinions on how to meet operational goals and efficiencies to achieve consensus. On-site employees often know as much as or more than paid consultants. They will help the institution meet its goals if they are asked for their help.
4. If the administrative team needs to make difficult decisions, it must appear fair and unbiased in its approach.
5. To be effective, the benchmarks and measurement tools used must be the same across the board for all staff at all levels of the organization.

6. If tough decisions need to be made, clear declarative statements should be given, with adequate warning. Allowing time for rumors to circulate may damage staff morale and disrupt the overall mission.
7. A formal approach to employee transition typically requires the assistance of human resources to ensure that the correct procedures and protocols are followed.
8. For cases that are more complicated or those involving a violation of policy or procedures regarding the transition process, legal counsel should be sought.
9. Self-awareness is maximized by using the 360-degree evaluation tool. For this tool to assess one's own performance accurately, it must truly be anonymous; however, most employees are wary about using a computerized entry system to provide feedback to their supervisors. The key is for administrators to establish rapport with staff, as well as trust and confidence in the corporate mission, by setting a good leadership example.

TABLE A.5. Keys to a successful administration–staff interface.

1. Remember that employee buy-in is key
2. Sell employees on the ideology
3. Ask employees for their opinions to achieve consensus
4. Use a fair and unbiased approach when making difficult decisions
5. Apply uniform benchmarking to all employee decisions
6. Ensure that communication is clear and timely
7. Enlist the support of human resources to ensure compliance
8. Consult legal counsel for more complicated cases
9. Encourage self-awareness feedback via a 360-degree assessment tool

Case 6: "Broke Another Instrument" (Surgeon Damaging Equipment)

Situation

The tales were legion at the hospital, especially in the operating suite. He had been there forever, or so it seemed. He was the only specialty surgeon in the area and had been a huge contributor to the hospital's vision and mission. Many trainees who rotated with this surgeon offered glowing recommendations of him based on his manner with patients and his surgical skill and clinical outcomes.

One major issue, however, had persisted through the years. The OR staff was always wary and on edge when working in this surgeon's operating suite, especially with regard to his treatment of surgical equipment. The typical scenario was triggered by the presence of a piece of equipment that was older, in disrepair, or substituting for the surgeon's preferred instrument. What followed was fairly routine for this provider; he usually destroyed the instrument or discarded it with significant fanfare. Sometimes, he pried the instrument apart first and then tossed the parts into the scrub bucket with quite a clatter. Usually, this behavior was accompanied by a diatribe concerning the hospital's cost-cutting initiatives and their adverse impact on his practice.

Although the OR staff generally were supportive—they had been adversely affected by these cutbacks as well—the surgeon's theatrics made some of them uncomfortable, and they felt his behavior was inappropriate in the workplace. Others felt that his destruction of equipment was a waste of scant resources and that he should be a leader and set an example for other health-care providers.

The surgeon's colleagues were sympathetic, as he often mirrored their sentiments and concerns as well. However, some of them felt that the issue of substandard equipment would be addressed better by a surgical committee or through discussions with the service-line director or the administrative team. They felt overwhelmed by their job responsibilities and did not want to be burdened with their colleague's disruptive behavior as well.

After the arm on an expensive surgical microscope was broken in the surgeon's OR suite, the biomedical department filed a complaint against him. Although no one actually witnessed the event, the surgeon previously made a reference to the device and his displeasure with it.

Issue

This scenario illustrates a surgeon's inappropriate behavior regarding hospital supplies and equipment and how all members of his OR team were involved.

Approach

In any day-to-day hospital operation, problems will arise regarding staff, supplies, or equipment. The method by which these problems are addressed is what determines success or failure.

1. Administration should ensure that proper equipment is available for staff use (Table A.6).
2. A multidisciplinary team involving nurses, technicians, and biomedical engineers is helpful in determining how to correct the behavior.
3. A mechanism should be in place to solicit and provide appropriate feedback concerning equipment. This groundwork will eliminate any subsequent rationale for inappropriate behavior.

4. At the first hint of destructive or abusive behavior, the involved party should be isolated and counseled concerning this behavior.

5. A zero-tolerance policy should be established for property abuse or destruction.

6. An incident report should be filed in anticipation of any future liability issues.

7. The provider should undergo a formal review and receive an action plan to prevent future events.

8. Depending on the nature of the incident and the costs incurred, law enforcement may need to be involved.

9. These situations often require psychotherapy, medication, and professionally orchestrated assistance groups.

10. The clearest initiative is to stop this behavior as soon as it occurs, before it spreads like a contagion throughout the system. Frustrations exist in all health-care systems; it is the responsibility of those in positions of authority to set a good example for all staff involved in the health-care delivery process.

TABLE A.6. Dealing with property abuse or destruction.

1. Ensure that proper equipment is available and working
2. Build a multidisciplinary focus team including biomedical engineers
3. Provide a mechanism for feedback
4. Isolate the first incident
5. Institute a zero-tolerance policy for property destruction
6. File an incident report in anticipation of liability
7. Conduct a formal review and provide an action plan
8. Consult law enforcement depending on the severity of the issue and cost of equipment lost
9. Recommend counseling, psychotherapy, or medication as needed

Case 7: "Called Off Again" (Physician Absenteeism)

Situation

You receive a panicked phone call from the department secretary. One of your partner physicians did not show up for her shift again. The night physician is still there, and the secretary wants to know how soon you can be there. You arrive within half an hour and relieve the night-shift physician.

The physician's absenteeism had become increasingly problematic, with a disproportionate number of absentee events attributed to her. On one event, she apologized over the phone, stating that she "had the flu" and that it wouldn't happen again. During the next few months, she called off two more times and was placed on probation and given an action plan.

Subsequently, the hospital instituted a new policy regarding changes in physicians' coverage responsibilities. On the day the changes took effect, she called off once again. This was construed as her not being supportive or accepting of the new policy.

Issue

Most hospital-based units run a fairly tight coverage schedule, and a provider calling off from work may be problematic. Among the nursing staff, employee call-offs are an expected part of the operation in some work environments. However, in some units, such as the ED or ICU, only one physician may be working per shift, and if that doctor is absent, the entire department may come to a standstill, which may be catastrophic to the patient care operation.

Approach

1. It must be determined whether staffing is adequate and appropriate for the clinical circumstances at hand (Table A.7).

2. A written policy should be instituted to deal with call-offs as they occur to minimize any adverse effects on patient are.

3. Another policy should be established to deal specifically with the expectations, requirements, and disciplinary issues related to work absenteeism.

4. The continuum may begin with a provider repeatedly calling off and progress to his or her failing to showing up for work without any notification.

5. The provider should be counseled early and decisively concerning his or her work attendance, requirements, and obligations.

6. The repercussions of any future variance from the protocol should be discussed.

7. Formal documentation of the discussion often is helpful in times of legal conflict.

8. The human resources team should standardize call-off protocols, so they are uniform throughout all hospital departments.

9. However, these protocols should account for differences based on unit, job description, and responsibilities, although they should be consistent within service lines.

10. A policy of requiring a physician to arrange for his or her own coverage often eliminates chronic absenteeism. The peer pressure of having to find another physician to cover one's shift is effective in minimizing repetitive call-off behavior.

11. The "no-show" provider presents a larger problem, and an external coverage system is still required.

12. Typically, a second no-show event should trigger an external investigation to determine whether substance abuse or behavioral issues are present.

The key is to establish reasonable, consistent expectations and to enforce them uniformly for the program to have external validity.

TABLE A.7. Dealing with habitual work absenteeism.

1. Ensure adequate staffing
2. Institute a written clinical policy
3. Make sure that the policy covers expectations, requirements, and disciplinary issues
4. Recognize the continuum from repeated "call-offs" to "no-show"
5. Counsel early and decisively
6. Discuss the repercussions of future policy violations
7. Document this discussion
8. Work with human resources to standardize protocols
9. Provide flexibility based on unit, job description, and responsibilities
10. Require providers to arrange their own coverage when calling off
11. Maintain an external coverage system for no-shows
12. Assess for behavioral problems or substance use

Case 8: "Out Late Again" (Substance Use by Resident)

Situation

The resident performed very well in the clinical workspace. He was bright, hardworking, and earnest. The staff found him easy to work with, and he was always available to them when they called. The patients also seemed to like him, and they often complimented him on his bedside manner and competence.

About halfway through the academic year, however, things started to change. The resident began to arrive late for his shift, and 1 day he did not show up at all. His work relationships were becoming strained as well, and he seemed to be a bit more irritable. At one point, he entered the wrong dose of a medication. Fortunately, one of the nurses caught the error and amended the order. The resident's excuse was that he had been up all night on call.

One of the attending physicians also noticed the changes in the resident's behavior. The resident's academic performance had declined, and he received the lowest in-service exam score for the group. In addition, questions were being raised about his performance during his clinical rotations.

There was talk about the resident staying out late and drinking heavily. At a recent residents' night out, he was grossly intoxicated. Even some of his fellow residents commented that they thought things were getting out of hand. Initially, they found his behavior amusing but then became increasingly concerned about it. Then photos were posted on social media showing the resident in a compromising position, appearing quite intoxicated, and involved in other inappropriate activities.

Previously, the resident had attended an informal counseling session during which he denied having a problem. However, this time a formal intervention was initiated, and the resident was put on probation. He was interviewed by a faculty panel and offered peer-to-peer support and professional counseling to address his substance use and work-related stressors.

Issue

Disruptive behavior often is precipitated by work-related stressors, such as high workload and expectations, as well as substance use or misuse. Although these problems may arise at any point in a physician's career, they tend to occur more frequently during early training.

Approach

1. Standard guidelines and regulations regarding physician training should be followed with regard to monitoring workload and other stressors (Table A.8).
2. A stress management program should be offered, with the option of outside confidential counseling if needed.
3. Behavioral expectations during training should be set and clearly defined from the outset.
4. A peer-to-peer network should be established to allow early intervention if possible.
5. An informal intervention should be offered as a first step to discuss guidelines and consequences.
6. The second event, or the first event if severe, should be addressed with a formal action plan.

7. The intervention may include direct supervision, work restriction, probation, or expulsion from the program.
8. A multidisciplinary faculty review panel may be helpful in performing the analysis and developing interventional strategies.
9. Some interventions may trigger a medical staff privilege or databank reporting requirement.
10. If any external sanctions are invoked, legal counsel should be consulted to establish the proper pathway and protocol for reporting.
11. Post-event counseling should be offered to establish positive behavioral coping strategies and healthy growth plans.
12. Reexamination should be performed periodically to monitor contract adherence, suitability for practice, or the need for practice restriction.
13. Referral to and participation in a state-based physician support and wellness program may improve the provider's adherence to the plan.

TABLE A.8. Monitoring behavioral issues during physician training.

1. Follow external training guidelines regarding workload
2. Provide a stress management program that allows for external consultation if needed
3. Define expectations regarding behavior during training
4. Institute a peer-to-peer early intervention program
5. As a first-step intervention, have a discussion with the physician regarding the guidelines and the consequences of violating them
6. Execute a formal action plan for a second event or a severe first event
7. Require intervention including direct supervision, work restriction, probation, or program expulsion
8. Review violations with a multidisciplinary faculty panel
9. Trigger medical staff privilege or databank reporting
10. Seek legal counsel if external sanctions are involved
11. Require post-event counseling for positive coping strategies
12. Reassess periodically for contract adherence and practice suitability
13. Refer the physician to a well-being program

Case 9: "I Am Not Taking That Admission" (Repeated Failure to Admit Patients)

Situation

The ED was literally packed with patients, meaning the rest of the hospital likely was full as well. Six patients were now waiting to be admitted. The hospitalist was called several times, but she did not answer the phone or return the calls. The charge nurse lamented that this particular physician "doesn't want to admit anyone; these patients will be here all night." The unit secretary chimed in, "She never calls back. I have to page her a half-dozen times to get a call."

Finally, the hospitalist responds, and the secretary puts the call through to you. You present the following case: "The patient is a 68-year-old female with hypertension, diabetes, and elevated cholesterol. She takes a regular aspirin daily. She had substernal chest pain that began yesterday, accompanied by shortness of breath and nausea...."

The hospitalist cuts you short saying, "Just send her home." You respond that the patient is high risk, with a high-risk presentation. She asks whether you can send a second cardiac enzyme, and you respond that she has a thrombolysis in myocardial infarction (TIMI) score of 3, prohibiting a rapid rule-out protocol.

"Well, what about a stress test?" asks the hospitalist. You reply that you tried to have one performed, but the echocardiographic department was closing for the day. "Well, I am not admitting her," she states emphatically. "Why don't you wait until morning, check another enzyme, and stress her then?" You tell her you will figure something out.

After a call to the patient's primary care provider and then her cardiologist, the patient was admitted. By that point, the house supervisor was involved and registered a concern about this admission practice that adversely affected the department's efficiency. This seemed to be a repetitive problem with the hospitalist's admission process.

Issue

The hospital admission process is one of great controversy as financial and efficiency demands increase at each facility. Opinions range from "we admit too many patients" to "the admission process makes it too difficult to get patients admitted."

Approach

1. To facilitate problem solving, the behavior should be classified correctly (Table A.9).
2. When clinical situations like this arise, the focus should always stay on the patients.
3. Any alleged disruptive behavior should be examined objectively by a third party.
4. The analysis should be completed by a practicing peer provider.
5. This process should involve the assistance of a case manager or other process analyst.
6. Peer or benchmark data should be used for reference when making comparisons.
7. An arbitration process, typically involving the nursing administrator on duty, should be used for contemporaneous problem resolution.
8. The medical staff hierarchy, including the department chairman and medical staff president, should be involved in the process to mediate and to enforce clinical compliance.
9. Continuing education should be provided to medical staff to help them keep abreast of changing admission policies. New guidelines and protocols seem to be generated daily.
10. The goals of any informal or formal remediation program should include ensuring proper standards of care.
11. The aforementioned programs should include training in negotiation, conflict resolution, and team building.

TABLE A.9. Handling differences of opinion in clinical care.

1. Classify behavior correctly to facilitate problem solving
2. Maintain a patient-centered focus
3. Seek third-party assessment of behavior
4. Arrange for practicing peer provider analysis
5. Ask a case manager or process analyst for assistance
6. Reference peer or benchmark data
7. Initiate arbitration for a contemporaneous resolution
8. Involve medical staff chairman and president
9. Provide continuing education on clinical process
10. Ensure an informal and a formal remediation process
11. Offer training in negotiation, conflict resolution, and team building

Case 10: "Suspended Again" (Persistent Failure to Complete Medical Records)

Situation

She was known throughout the institution as a wonderful physician. She had good clinical acumen and a nice bedside manner, and she worked well with the staff. However, she had one persistent, noticeable problem: her documentation and medical record completion rate was poor compared with that of her peers. There were significant delays in all aspects of her medical record documentation, as well as inaccuracies in her patients' records. The deficiencies seemed to be pervasive.

The facility had an electronic health records program, and it still used a traditional paper chart system to record some aspects of patient information. It followed conventional guidelines for accuracy, validity, and timeliness in completing medical records. Nevertheless, the physician had not completed her patients' records for some time. Although the medical records department tried to accommodate her many requests for additional time, her compliance never seemed to improve.

The physician had had several recent suspensions, and an action plan was in place for one last attempt at medical record completion compliance for this individual. Moreover, the medical records department was preparing for an upcoming visit by the Joint Commission to ensure the facility was in compliance regarding recordkeeping. Records staff attempted to contact the physician to complete additional required dictations, amend missing documents, and include electronic signatures on completed records. She responded a few days after the deadline, stating she had been on vacation.

Issue

Universally accepted guidelines exist regarding both accuracy and timeliness in completing medical records. For surgical cases, history and physical examination findings must be documented within 24 h. Overall, federal guidelines require medical records to be completed within 30 days, but some states mandate that recordkeeping be completed within as little as 15 days.

Approach

1. It is essential to establish and then educate providers on conventionally accepted standards of performance (Table A.10).
2. A process also should be delineated whereby a provider can compare his or her compliance to the established standards.
3. A plan should be developed and executed to notify physicians about the requirements for successfully completing the tasks at hand.
4. The hospital's remediation plan for noncompliance with time-sensitive regulatory requirements should be clearly defined.
5. Multiple secure communication approaches should be available to physicians to facilitate their compliance with documentation. Programs that offer only one unnecessarily rigid route to compliance may limit their success.
6. Hiring an administrative assistant to assist with documentation tasks may be considered as a last ditch effort to avoid care exclusion.
7. A discussion should be held with the physician regarding all aspects of documentation, including quality and the

medicolegal and financial consequences of suboptimal or
untimely documentation.

8. Written notice with a trackable remediation plan should
   be provided to noncompliant physicians.
9. A program of escalating interventions should be instituted, beginning with suspension of admitting privileges
   and ending with loss of medical staff privileges.
10. Any remediation or punitive intervention should be dis-
    cussed with and approved by the department chair and
    then by the medical staff president.
11. All measures should be attempted to resolve the problem
    internally before a report is submitted to an outside agency.
12. Follow-up meetings should be held and a behavioral con-
    tract should be drafted and signed by all parties involved
    to document the appropriate path to correction.
13. Hospital compliance must be maintained, even if that
    requires a personnel change.

TABLE A.10. Tips to ensure compliance with medical records
requirements.

1. Establish standards of performance and educate staff on them
2. Delineate a process for a provider to gauge his or her
   compliance with the established standards
3. Institute a system for informing providers about requirements
4. Define a remediation plan for violating time-sensitive hospital
   requirements
5. Ensure multiple secure communication routes to achieve
   compliance
6. Hire an administrative assistant to help with documentation
7. Discuss quality and medicolegal and financial impacts of
   noncompliance
8. Provide written notice with a trackable remediation plan
9. Use escalating interventions from admitting privilege
   suspension to loss of medical staff privileges
10. Discuss remediation with department chair and medical staff
    president
11. Maximize internal measures before resorting to external ones
12. Follow up with a behavioral contract
13. Maintain hospital compliance at all costs

Index

© Springer International Publishing Switzerland 2016
R.B. Vukmir, *Disruptive Healthcare Provider Behavior*,
DOI 10.1007/978-3-319-27924-4

Printed in the United States
By Bookmasters